IFMBE Proceedings

Volume 50

The International Federation for Medical and Biological Engineering, IFMBE, is a federation of national and transnational organizations representing internationally the interests of medical and biological engineering and sciences. The IFMBE is a non-profit organization fostering the creation, dissemination and application of medical and biological engineering knowledge and the management of technology for improved health and quality of life. Its activities include participation in the formulation of public policy and the dissemination of information through publications and forums. Within the field of medical, clinical, and biological engineering, IFMBE's aims are to encourage research and the application of knowledge, and to disseminate information and promote collaboration. The objectives of the IFMBE are scientific, technological, literary, and educational.

The IFMBE is a WHO accredited NGO covering the full range of biomedical and clinical engineering, healthcare, healthcare technology and management. It is representing through its 60 member societies some 120.000 professionals involved in the various issues of improved health and health care delivery.

More information about this series at http://www.springer.com/series/7403

Ákos Jobbágy
Editor

First European Biomedical Engineering Conference for Young Investigators

ENCY2015, Budapest, May 28-30, 2015

Springer

Editor

Ákos Jobbágy
Department of Measurement and Information Systems
Budapest University of Technology and Economics (BME)
Budapest
Hungary

ISSN 1680-0737 ISSN 1433-9277 (electronic)
IFMBE Proceedings
ISBN 978-981-287-572-3 ISBN978-981-287-573-0 (eBook)
DOI 10.1007/978-981-287-573-0

Library of Congress Control Number: 2015941124

Springer Singapore Heidelberg New York Dordrecht London

The IFMBE Proceedings is an Official Publication of the International Federation for Medical and Biological Engineering (IFMBE)

Printed on acid-free paper

Springer is part of Springer Science+Business Media (www.springer.com)

Preface

Does it make sense to organize a conference for young investigators? What are its specialties?

Based on my experience the research activity of young guys is strong enough, their papers are well written (usually helped by senior colleagues). They are not so good at making oral presentations and are lacking travel funds.

The First European Biomedical Conference for Young Investigators - ENCY - tries to accommodate for these specialties. The scientific level for accepting a paper was kept high; you can check it in the proceedings. Participants even in the early phase of their scientific career have been given the chance to hold a lecture about their research work. The audience is supposed to be sympathetic being composed of mainly young ones. Nevertheless, a few professors provide help by holding invited lectures and chairing the sessions.

The cost of attending ENCY was kept extremely low - as low as possible. Organizers have been volunteering, Budapest University of Technology and Economics provided the room and audiovisual facilities free of charge, cheap accommodation was provided.

We hope ENCY will continue. In every two years a biomedical engineering research group in Europe will take the responsibility to organize the event!

Budapest
May 2015

Ákos Jobbágy
conference chair

Organization

International Program Committee

Péter Antal
Joe Barbanel
Ferenc Bari
Zoltán Benyó
Imre Bojtár
Tamás Dabóczi
Sergo Dadunashvili
Yuri Dekhtyar
László Dézsi
Ferenc Ender
Jiří Holčík
Timo Jämsä
Tomaž Jarm
Miklós Kellermayer
Rita Kiss
Jordan Kolev
Levente Kovács
Igor Lackovič
Dávid Légrády
Lenka Lhotska
Olof Lindahl
Ratko Magjarevič
Kalju Meigas
Nicolas Pallikarakis
Leandro Pecchia
Krzysztof Penkala
Laura Roa
Karel Roubik
Andres Santos
Armen Sargsyan
Pál Simon
Rita Stagni
András Szarka
Heikki Teriö

Table of Contents

Genomic Approach to Complex Diseases

Csaba Szalai

Semmelweis University, Department of Genetics, Cell and Immunobiology and Heim Pál Hospital; Budapest, Hungary

Abstract- **The complex or multifactorial diseases are those which develop through interactions of often hundreds of genes and environmental factors. The complex diseases like cancer, asthma, hypertension, diabetes mellitus, cardiovascular diseases or Alzheimer disease are often very frequent, it can even be said that more or less everybody is affected by some of them. In this review it is discussed why it is important to study the genomic background of the complex diseases and the main genomic methods are summarized. Next, the difficulties of these studies are shown and discussed what the reason of the missing heritability of the complex diseases can be. In the end some developments are shown which try to cope with these problems.**

Keywords- **multifactorial diseases, genetic markers, genetic variants, genomic methods, missing heritability.**

I. Introduction

The complex or multifactorial diseases are those which develop through interactions of a few (oligogenic) or several (polygenic) genes and the environmental factors. The complex diseases, in contrast to the monogenic diseases, which affect only a small fraction of the population, are often very frequent, it can even be said that more or less everybody is affected by them. Complex diseases are the endemic, non-communicable diseases, or NCD, which are non-infectious and non-transmissible between persons, like cancer, asthma, hypertension, diabetes mellitus, cardiovascular diseases and Alzheimer disease, etc.

First, one can ask, why it is important to study the genomic background of the complex diseases? Perhaps the most important is that it helps to explore the molecular pathomechanism. In contrast to the traditional methods, the genomic methods are often hypothesis free, i.e. they do not require any knowledge about the pathogenesis. In this way novel pathways and mechanisms can be detected, which can offer new drug targets or new therapies. Otherwise, the genomic studies can reveal the genetic differences between people, offering novel possibilities for personal therapies, and connections can be found between the success of the therapy and the genetic background. Genomic studies can reveal genetic variations which influence the risk of developing a disease. In this way, right after the birth the genomic background and the risk to different diseases of a new-born can be determined, which offers the possibilities to change from "diagnose and treat" to "predict and prevent". Earlier it was regarded as the most important task of the medical genomics, but later it turned out that in most cases the sum risk to a multifactorial disease is so complex that it is usually impossible to give a clinically relevant estimation.

As for both researchers and the whole society the significance of genomic results are widespread appreciated, this has led to a large-scale effort for the development of genomic methods and huge breakthroughs have been achieved.

II. Genomic Studies

A. Genetic markers

A genetic marker is usually a sequence variation with a known location on a chromosome that can be used to identify individuals, with a relative high chance to differentiate between different alleles on homologous chromosomes. Genetic markers can be used to study the relationship between an inherited disease and its genetic cause (for example, a particular mutation of a gene that results in a defective protein). It is known that pieces of DNA that lie near each other on a chromosome tend to be inherited together (they are linked). This property enables the use of a marker, which can then be used to determine the precise inheritance pattern of the gene that has not yet been exactly localized. Genetic markers have to be easily identifiable, associated with a specific locus, and highly polymorphic, because homozygotes do not provide any information.

One of the most popular markers are the microsatellites, or simple sequence repeats (SSRs) or short tandem repeats (STRs), are repeating sequences of 2-6 base pairs of DNA. Often they are very polymorphic, meaning that individuals are often heterozygotic to them, which means that they differ in the number of repeats.

They are widely used in mapping disease genes or differentiate between individuals. The human genome is now mapped by approximately 30,000 highly polymorphic microsatellites. The average length of linkage disequilibrium (LD) for microsatellites is ~100 kb, which is considerably higher than that of SNPs. Therefore, a single microsatellite captures a larger genomic region than does a single SNP. Microsatellites also provide several other advantages, such as a higher information content (6–10 alleles as compared with 2 alleles for SNPs), and a smaller interpopulation variability. Most existing forensic DNA databases are STR-based. It has been demonstrated that 20–50 ascertained autosomal SNPs could reach match probabilities similar to those obtained with 10–15 forensically used STRs.

But the disadvantages of the STRs are that the detection methods are quite complicated relative to those of the SNPs,

Á. Jobbágy (ed.), *First European Biomedical Engineering Conference for Young Investigators*,
IFMBE Proceedings 50, DOI: 10.1007/978-981-287-573-0_1

they are much rarer than SNPs, and their mutation rates are 100,000 times higher.
Nowadays, the advantages of the SNPs are much more significant, and mainly because of their number and simple detection techniques, they will replace STRs in most areas. E.g. forty-five unlinked autosomal SNPs were ascertained by screening more than 500 candidate SNPs in 44 worldwide populations. These 45 ascertained SNPs have high levels of heterozygosity and low levels of population differentiation and are therefore suitable for universal human identification purposes. Multiplex genotyping assays for these SNPs have been developed.

B. *Study of genetic variants*

Genetic variations play important roles in disease susceptibilities, differences between individuals or in responses to drugs, and the study of them is important in discovery of novel drug targets, personal therapies or pharmacogenetics, etc. The HGP and the subsequent different genome projects (Human Variome Project, HapMap, 1000 Genome project, etc.) detected millions of genetic variants [1,2]. Presently, there are more than 65 million short variants, and more than 10 million structural variants in the databases.
The simplest method for the study of the genetic background of a disease is the candidate gene association study. In these studies genes are selected, which are thought to play a role in the disease. Then, genetic variations are searched in these genes. Earlier the genes were sequenced in several individuals, now the databases contain practically all the common variants. The first one is often called wet laboratory method, the latter one *in silico* method. Then, the selected variants are genotyped, and their frequencies are compared in the population with and without the studied trait (disease). If the frequencies of the variants differ in a statistically significant way between the two populations, then they are suspected to play a role in the disease susceptibility. Several 10 thousand such investigations have been carried out in the last decades in different diseases. But, there were a lot of problems with these studies. One of the problems is the multiple testing problems, but in a different way than discussed in connection with GWAS (s. later). Because here, the same variants have been tested in different laboratories, and naturally only the positive results have been published; the negative ones have been discarded. And, if 100 laboratories study the same variants, there is a chance that one of them gets a positive association purely by chance. This is called publication bias. Because of this, hundreds of false positive results (and genes) have been published.
The other problem is that with this methods only those genes can be studied whose role was already known in the disease, and in this way no new mechanism could be detected.
The hypothesis-free genomic methods theoretically could solve this last problem. First, whole genome screenings were developed and carried out in several diseases. In this method families were screened with microsatellites. Those families were recruited where there were at least two affected siblings. These studies are also called affected sib pair (ASP) studies, or linkage studies. Here LOD scores were calculated. The LOD score (logarithm (base 10) of odds) is a statistical test often used for linkage analysis. The LOD score compares the likelihood of obtaining the test data if the two loci, or the disease phenotype and a locus are indeed linked, to the likelihood of observing the same data purely by chance. Positive LOD scores favor the presence of linkage, whereas negative LOD scores indicate that linkage is less likely. A LOD score greater than 3.0 is considered evidence for linkage. A LOD score of +3 indicates 1000 to 1 odds that the linkage being observed did not occur by chance. On the other hand, a LOD score of less than -2.0 is considered evidence to exclude linkage.
The method has given a lot of interesting results, but there have been several problems with it. First, it is difficult to collect families with two affected siblings, second, the genotyping of the microsatellies are very cumbersome and expensive. Because of this latter, the number of microsatellites in the studies was limited (usually not more than 400), thus the resolution was very low. This means that it was a great chance that disease associated loci, which were not in linkage with any of the microsatellites were lost. In addition, these studies could determine only genomic regions (because of the limited number of markers), and not genes. And often, these regions are large, several megabase long and contain several hundreds of genes. In this way, additional methods are needed for the determination of the genes.

C. *GWAS*

Presently, the most popular method for the study of the genomic background of complex diseases and traits is called GWAS (genome-wide association study), also known as whole genome association study (WGA study or WGAS). The method has become possible, when arrays and chips have been developed with which first 100 thousand, then several million SNP could be genotyped in one measurement, and the price of one chip has become relatively cheap, i.e. about $100. First, only SNPs were determined, later, when the significance of CNVs became apparent, they were involved as well. The CNVs were determined through their known linkage with SNPs. In 2007 this method was selected for the breakthrough of the year.
There are two main companies in the markets, Affymetrix and Illumina. The Affymetrix Genome-Wide Human SNP Array 6.0 features 1.8 million genetic markers, including more than 906,600 SNPs and more than 946,000 probes for the detection of CNVs.
The Illumina HumanOmni5-Quad (Omni5) BeadChip can detect 4.3 million tagSNPs selected from the International HapMap and 1000 Genomes Projects that target genetic variation down to 1% minor allele frequency (MAF).
In GWAS the distribution (frequencies) of the variants is compared in the different populations; usually one of them is affected with the trait, the other is not. But, with the development of the statistical methods GWAS has become capable of studying the genomic background of continuous

traits (like fasting glucose levels or blood pressure) as well. In this latter case there are no different groups.

GWAS has been offering a great chance for the investigation of the genomic background of the diseases, which have been utilized by a lot of research groups and consortia. Because of the strict statistical conditions and the large investigated populations, the results of GWAS may contain only few false results; and because this is a hypothesis-free method, there is a possibility that it reveals new aspects of the disease. To make these important results public, a web page was established on 25 November 2008 (A Catalog of Published Genome-Wide Association Studies) [3], and it includes only those publications which investigate at least 100,000 SNPs in the initial stage. Publications are organized from most to least recent date of publication, indexing from online publication if available. Studies focusing only on candidate genes are excluded from this catalog. Studies are identified through weekly PubMed literature searches, daily NIH-distributed compilations of news and media reports, and occasional comparisons with an existing database of GWAS. SNP-trait associations listed here are limited to those with p-values < 1.0 × 10-5. In 2013 the catalog contained about 1,800 curated publications of 12,000 SNPs [4]. In March 2015, the GWAS Catalog infrastructure was migrating to the European Bioinformatics Institute (EMBL-EBI).

D. Evaluation of GWAS results

The evaluation and handling of GWAS data are a great challenge for the bioinformaticians. One of the main problems is the multiple testing problem. If the p value of a SNP corresponds to the Bonferroni corrected value, then it is said that it reached the level of genome wide significance. It is, e.g. in case of 1 million SNPs 5×10^{-8}. As the main characteristics of the complex diseases are variants with weak effects, this low p value often can only be achieved through involving large populations. Often the number of participants must be >100,000, which is very difficult and expensive to collect, and which is in case of rarer diseases even impossible. Because of this, GWAS are often carried out by large international consortia.

A method to attenuate this problem can be, if several smaller populations are investigated independently. In this way the p values in the independent studies for each SNP are multiplied, and it is easier to achieve the low values (e.g. $10^{-3} \times 10^{-3} = 10^{-6}$). Usually, a discovery GWAS is carried out in a smaller population (discovery cohort). Then, SNPs are selected with a not so strict p value (e.g. cut off value $< 5\times 10^{-2}$), then several independent populations are collected (replication cohorts), and only the selected SNPs are studied. The SNPs which are confirmed in the replication cohorts can be those which are associated with the disease.

New statistical methods are also under development, such as Bayesian statistics and pathway analysis. For this latter, several databases are available like Gene Ontology (GO) [5] or KEGG (Kyoto Encyclopedia of Genes and Genomes [6].

Gene Set Enrichment Analysis (GSEA) is a computational method, which was originally developed for gene expression studies and can be applied in GWAS as well. This determines whether different a priori defined sets of genes show statistically significant, concordant differences between two biological states (e.g. phenotypes). Then the sets of genes are ranked according to their associations.

With these methods several new disease associated pathways have been detected.

E. DNA sequencing

DNA sequencing is the process of reading the nucleotide bases in a DNA molecule. Since the beginning of the HGP it has been developing continuously. In HGP the DNA was sequenced with Sanger method, i.e. with dideoxy or chain termination sequencing. In 2001 the sequencing of one human genome took a minimum of 1 year. It was obvious that both the price and the time were not appropriate for routine investigations, or even for sequencing several human genomes. It became clear that the Sanger method could not be developed much further to become much cheaper and faster. But it was also obvious that much cheaper and faster sequencing would have an immense leap in pharmaceutical research, personal medicine, but it could be used for countless aims. The high demand for low-cost sequencing has driven the development of high-throughput sequencing (also called as next-generation sequencing, or NGS) technologies that parallelize the sequencing process, producing thousands or millions of sequences at once. The methods were so successful that in 2007 the new generation sequencing (NGS) became the method of the year [7] in *Nature Methods* magazine. In 2007 the genome of James Watson was sequence with the 454 technology in 2 months and for $1 million. It was still far away from the aim, but it was a big step ahead. Since then, the price has been lower and lower, and the time shorter and shorter (Figure 2). E.g. in June 2009, Illumina announced that they were launching their own Personal Full Genome Sequencing Service at a depth of 30× for US $48,000 per genome.

In November 2009, Complete Genomics published a peer-reviewed paper in *Science* demonstrating its ability to sequence a complete human genome for US$1,700. If true, this would mean the cost of full genome sequencing has come down exponentially within just a single year from around US$100,000 to US$50,000 and now to US$1,700.

In 2011 Complete Genomics charges approximately US$10,000 to sequence a complete human genome (less for large orders).

In May 2011, Illumina lowered its Full Genome Sequencing service to US$5,000 per human genome, or US$4,000 if ordering 50 or more.

In January 2012, Life Technologies introduced a sequencer to decode a human genome in one day for $1,000 and now several examples of other equipment are also capable for this.

F. Difficulties in the studies of the genomic background of complex diseases

At the beginning of the genomic era, even right after the completion of the HGP, it was generally thought that genomic would revolutionize the medicine, and in a few years the era of personal therapy would come. But now we know that it did not come true, and even it would not in the next years. What can be the reason for this?

According to the general opinion, one of the main reasons for this failure is due to the very complex regulation of the genome, and the multifactorial nature of the diseases and traits. In Table 1 there are some characteristics which make the determination of the genetic background of the multifactorial diseases difficult.

Table 1 Factors, which make the determination of the genetic backgrounds of the complex diseases difficult

Problems	Explanation
Genetic heterogeneity	Different allelic combinations lead to similar phenotypes.
Phenocopy	Environmental factors lead to the same clinical phenotype as do the genetic factors. In other words, the environmental condition mimics the phenotype produced by a gene.
Pleiotropy	The genetic variation can lead to different phenotypes.
Incomplete penetrance	Some individuals fail to express the trait, even though they carry the trait associated alleles.
The exact diagnosis is difficult	Often in complex diseases there are no standard diagnoses. There are subtypes of the diseases that cannot be differentiated with standard methods. The symptoms can change with the time, or manifest in episodes. Different diseases with similar symptoms. Concordance of different diseases.

As for both researchers and the whole society the significance of genomic results are widespread appreciated, this has led to a large-scale effort for the development of genomic methods and huge breakthroughs have been achieved.

But there is no reason for the total satisfaction, since most of the aims have not been achieved. In 2009, Manolio et al. published a widespread cited table in a paper, which summarizes the results of studies aiming at determining the genomic background of multifactorial diseases and traits [8]. These results show that the GWAS, which were thought to be the very method for determining the genomic background of complex traits, could determine only a small fraction of the heritability proportion of the majority of the traits. It means that most variants identified until then conferred relatively small increments in risk, and explained only a small proportion of familial clustering, leading many to question how the remaining, 'missing' heritability can be explained. And the situation has not improved considerably since then. E.g. height is one of the QTs which is easy to determine, and it is known that the heritability of it is about 80%. In several studies, large populations were collected and several GWAS were carried out. In one study, 44 loci were determined, which were responsible only for 5% of the heritability. Later, 180 loci could be determined, but they were still responsible only for 10% of the heritability. This is true for the majority of the diseases. E.g. this value for T2DM is 6%, for fasting glucose level is 1.5%, for early myocardial infarction is 2.8%. The exceptions are diseases, where there are only a couple of mutations with strong impact, like in the case of macular degeneration. In contrast, the determination of the genetic background of monogenic diseases is a great success; it has been clarified for about 4000 such diseases so far.

What can be the reason for this situation, which is often called the dark matter of heritability? Previously, some explanations have been already mentioned and below some additional ones will be given.

G. Problems of the rare variants

GWAS work with pre-made chips, which could determine known variations with a population frequency of >5% (MAF = minor allele frequency). There is a theory named common disease - common variants or CD/CV, which says that common diseases are caused by several common (frequent) variants with weak effects. The weak effects of these variants are accumulated causing higher susceptibility to a disease. If the environmental factors are unfavourable, then the disease can develop. It proved to be true for a lot of traits, like Alzheimer disease, where the roles of the common apoE4 variants or the obesity where the roles of variations in the FTO genes were verified. But, there are also proofs for the so-called common disease rare variants hypothesis (CD/RV), which states that the common diseases are caused by rare variants with strong effects [9]. Example is the breast cancer where thousands of rare variants with strong effects have been found. The rare variants cannot be determined with GWAS, and the traditional statistical methods are not suitable for their detection. It is suggested that even in diseases, where common variations are known, there are also rare variations with strong effect.

The rare variants can also cause another statistical problem called synthetic associations. In this case rare variants at the locus create multiple independent association signals captured by common tagging SNPs causing that variants which do not participate in the given phenotype, will be falsely named.

H. The random behavior of the genome

In September 2010 researchers published in Nature that genetic circuits that regulate cellular functions are subject to stochastic fluctuations, or 'noise', in the levels of their components [10]. It means that the behavior of the genome is sometimes random and thus cannot be predicted in 100%. It means that it is theoretically impossible even with more developed genomic and informatic methods to exactly forecast the future traits (phenotypes) of a newborn.

I. Statistical problems

The next problem originates from the evaluation methods, i.e. from the statistics. The most variations associated with increased risk to complex diseases, increase the risk with only 10-20%. It means that the chance in the carriers for the development of the disease is only 1.1-1.2 times higher than in non-carriers. Detecting variations with such weak effects is very difficult. In addition, as the population is genetically heterogeneous, and interactions between these variants are needed, the possible number of genetic backgrounds associated with increased risk is practically infinite. In statistical point of view it is advantageous if the population is larger, but the larger population is genetically more heterogeneous, thus the effect of each genetic variant is diluted, becoming less significant and may be lost.

The other problem is the lack of proper statistical methods. One problem is called the multiple testing problem.

If in a GWAS 100 thousand genetic variations are measured, in a statistical point of view it means that 100 thousand independent measurements are carried out. In this case the probabilities of the false results are summed up. In statistics, $p < 0.05$ is used as a significance threshold. It means that the probability of the false statement is 5% (we can make a false statement 5 times in 100 independent investigations). One of the methods to correct this is called Bonferroni correction. In this case, 0.05 is divided by the number of the measurements (in this case with 100 thousand; $p = 0.05/100.000 = 5\times10^{-7}$). But the number of the independent investigations depends not only on the number of the measurements, but on several other factors, like the number of the samples, the clinical parameters and the type of tests, etc. But the Bonferroni correction is too conservative, i.e. if the correction is applied, only the strongest effects can be detected. In contrast, according to the CD/CV hypothesis the complex diseases develop through interactions between multiple genetic variants with weak effects and the environment. In addition, as the genetic factors interact with each other, if we want to calculate this interaction as well, it would increase the number of independent questions to a very large number. It means that the Bonferroni corrections and the similar other methods are not capable of detecting the variants of weak effects, i.e. other methods are needed.

J. Possible solutions

There are several developments which try to cope with the above mentioned problems. E.g. utilizing the results of the 1000 Genome Project, new chips are under development, which can measure rarer (MAF < 0.05) variants as well (e.g. Illumina 5M chip). Furthermore, next to genotyping based methods, the new generation sequencing (NGS) may be soon suitable for population based studies. With the NGS, all type of variations can be detected. It must be added, however, that the statistical problems are even larger with this method, since it can give terabit size of data and hundreds of thousands of variations, many of which can be sequencing mistakes, or unknown variations whose functional characterizations are immensely difficult.

There are a couple of new solutions for the statistical problems as well. E.g. to overcome several of the limitations, probabilistic graphical models (PGMs) were proposed. Thanks to their ability to efficiently and accurately represent complex networks, PGMs represent powerful tools to dissect the genetic susceptibility of complex diseases. Bayesian networks are a popular class of PGMs, its graphical representation presents a crucial advantage and is able to efficiently deal with SNP–SNP interactions impacting the phenotype, a situation that is called epistasis. As Bayes statistics can evaluate networks, it is a suitable evaluation method for systems biology [11-13].

It is assumed that with better statistics significantly more information can be extracted even from the present results. E.g. in a paper it has been stated that from the old results but with better statistics they could explain 67% of the heritability of height, in contrast the 5% in the original paper. In this paper rather than considering SNPs one by one, the new statistical analysis considers what effect all the SNPs together have on height [14].

In another paper the genetic background of hypertension was studied. They reevaluated the results of a metaanalysis of several GWAS, which did not find any associated variants (owing to the too conservative Bonferroni correction, and the heterogeneous nature of this disease). In the new statistics the authors did not consider individual SNPs, but examined whether there are pathways where the distribution of the variations are statistically different in the hypertensive population relative to the controls. In this paper several pathways were found associated with the disease [15].

It is also a great challenge that the majority (~93%) of disease- and trait-associated variants emerging from these studies lie within non-coding sequence. It is therefore very difficult to explain how these variants influence the trait. In a study of the ENCODE project it was found that in a given cell line, 76.6% of all non-coding GWAS SNPs either lie within a DNase I hypersensitive site (DHS) (57.1% or 2931 SNPs), or are in complete linkage disequilibrium (LD) with SNPs in a nearby DHS [16]. DHSs show remarkable concordance with experimentally determined and computationally predicted binding sites of transcription factors and enhancers. With the help of the results of the ENCODE and similar other projects it will be much easier to determine the function of a variant lying in non-coding region of the genome.

Acknowledgment

This study was supported by OTKA (Hungarian Scientific Research Fund): K112872

Conflict of Interest

The author declares that he has no conflict of interest.

References

1. Venter JC, Adams MD, Myeers EW et al (2001) The sequence of the Human Genome. Science 291:1304-51

2. International Human Genome Sequencing Consortium (2004) Finishing the euchromatic sequence of the human genome Nature 431: 931 - 945
3. http://www.genome.gov/gwastudies/
4. Welter D, MacArthur J, Morales J et al. (2014) The NHGRI GWAS Catalog, a curated resource of SNP-trait associations. Nucleic Acids Res 42 (Database issue):D1001-6
5. http://www.geneontology.org
6. http://www.genome.jp/kegg/
7. http://www.nature.com/nmeth/journal/v5/n1/full/nmeth1157.html
8. Manolio TA, Collins FS, Cox NJ, et al. (2009) Finding the missing heritability of complex diseases. Nature 461(7265):747-53
9. McClellan J, King MC (2010) Genetic heterogeneity in human disease. Cell 141(2):210-7.
10. Eldar A, Elowitz MB (2010) Functional roles for noise in genetic circuits. Nature 467(7312):167-73.
11. Ungvári I, Hullám G, Antal P et al. (2012) Evaluation of a partial genome screening of two asthma susceptibility regions using Bayesian network based Bayesian multilevel analysis of relevance. PLoS One 7(3):e33573.
12. Lautner-Csorba O, Gézsi A, Semsei AF, et al. (2012) Candidate gene association study in pediatric acute lymphoblastic leukemia evaluated by Bayesian network based Bayesian multilevel analysis of relevance. BMC Med Genomics 5(1):42.
13. Lautner-Csorba O, Gézsi A, Erdélyi DJ et al. (2013) Roles of genetic polymorphisms in the folate pathway in childhood acute lymphoblastic leukemia evaluated by bayesian relevance and effect size analysis. PLoS One. 8(8):e69843.
14. Yang J, Benyamin B, McEvoy BP et al. (2010) Common SNPs explain a large proportion of the heritability for human height. Nat Genet 42(7):565-9.
15. Torkamani A, Topol EJ, Schork NJ (2008) Pathway analysis of seven common diseases assessed by genome-wide association. Genomics 92(5):265-72.
16. ENCODE Project Consortium (2012) An integrated encyclopedia of DNA elements in the human genome. Nature 489(7414):57-74.

Author address:
Author: Szalai Csaba
Institute: Semmelweis University, Department of Genetics, Cell and Immunobiology
Street: Nagyvárad tér 4.
City: Budapest
Country: Hungary
Email: szalaics@gmail.com

Modeling and Control of Physiological Systems

L. Kovacs

Obuda University, John von Neumann Faculty of Informatics, Physiological Controls Group, Budapest, Hungary

Abstract— **The aim of physiological modeling and control is to study, model and understand biological processes, then to apply identification and control strategies on it as a system. It is a big challenge to combine individualized control therapies with physiological model-based robust control methods. This requires a combination of mathematical knowledge (numeric-symbolic computations), control engineering (system identification, control theory), computer engineering (formal methods, software development and testing) and biomedical engineering (physiological modeling. The paper discusses current challenges of this topic by three concrete examples: diabetes, tumor control and depth of anesthesia.**

Keywords— **physiological modeling, control, artificial pancreas, tumor control, anesthesia.**

I. INTRODUCTION

Control engineering represents a major field in engineering, with great contribution to technological advancement. Control theory gives the background to control engineering that started evolving at the beginning of the 20th century. It first considered the analysis and control of linear systems, e.g. typical controller architectures and design methodologies of the 20th century, PID control, state-feedback controls, such as pole-placement or LQ control. Nowadays, the main trend in control sciences is still the development of linear controllers in an optimal and robust sense by using modern robust control techniques, like H_∞ control or μ-synthesis [1], based on linear system dynamics.

The technological advancement due to control theory has slowed down since the dynamical systems that are not under artificial control are usually nonlinear systems, ex. biomedical systems [2].

Since nonlinear dynamical systems represent a significantly greater family than linear dynamical systems, the control of nonlinear systems is much less elaborated than the control of linear ones. Existing nonlinear control techniques, like exact linearization through state-feedback [3], or linear parameter varying (LPV) based control basically reduce the nonlinear control problem to a linear one; however, higher computational power is needed [4].

Since control theory mostly consists of model-based design methodologies, acquiring the model of the system in question is a crucial task. The method that deals with system model acquisition is covered by system identification theory. System identification is a well elaborated [5], but still evolving field of control science and econometrics; however, the area of application is restricted to linear systems. Identification of nonlinear dynamical systems is still an open and important research problem.

In the biomedical research domain, experts typically face two major problems:

1) understanding the physiological behavior of the system and transform it into a (mathematical) model;
2) finding sufficiently accurate methods and sensory input modes to detect the required signals.

The aim of physiological modeling and control – a subdiscipline of biomedical engineering – is to study, model and understand biological processes, then to apply identification and control strategies on it as a system [6]. This approach enables the automated treatment of various diseases (ex. diabetes or cancer) and injuries of the human body (e.g. bio-prosthetics) by designing closed-loop control systems; hence, enabling personalized healthcare by giving the possibility to support medical devices for specific diseases or ease everyday life healthcare monitoring (i.e. by smartphone applications).

Using control engineering methodologies (model identification and controller design) these protocols could become model-based.

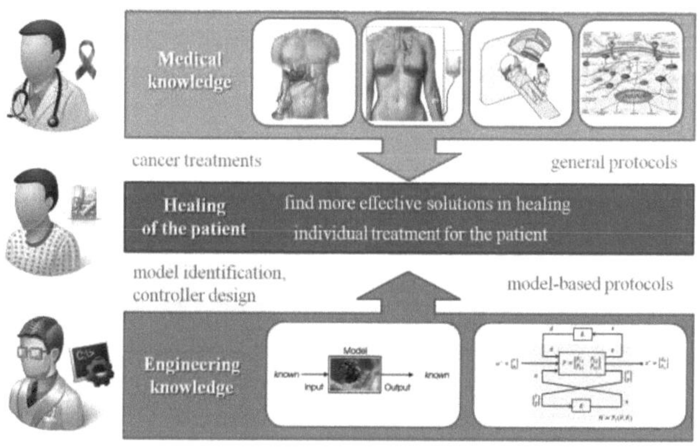

Fig. 1 Cancer treatments (surgical oncology, chemotherapy, radiotherapy and targeted molecular therapies) provide general protocols. Taking into account control engineering methodologies (model identification and controller design) the protocols could become model-based and the treatment could be personalized.

Á. Jobbágy (ed.), *First European Biomedical Engineering Conference for Young Investigators*,
IFMBE Proceedings 50, DOI: 10.1007/978-981-287-573-0_2

Model-based design allows finding more effective solutions in healing and individual treatment for the patient. The concept can be represented in Fig. 1 from cancer treatments point of view.

The paper highlights the context of current challenges of physiological modeling and control under three topics: diabetes, cancer and anesthesia; namely, the trade-off between guaranteeing robustness, but creating individualized / personalized control solutions as well.

II. DIABETES MODELING AND CONTROL: THE ARTIFICIAL PANCREAS PROBLEM

Diabetes mellitus is a serious metabolic disease that should be artificially regulated. Due to the continuously increasing number of diabetic patients, the scientific community has aimed to improve the treatment of the disease by investigating the applicability of an external controller, so called artificial pancreas [7] (AP) that focus on Type 1 Diabetes Models (T1DM) having a general clinical symptom, the lack of insulin production of the patients.

Since T1DM models have usually nonlinear dynamics [8], the controllers used for blood glucose regulation are either nonlinear as well, or linear while consider the nonlinearity of the model by giving robust guarantees. An example for the latter is robust H_∞ control [1]. Robustness is necessary, as classical linear control methods (e.g. PID control [9]) faces difficulties ensuring the safety of the patient, and hence has limited practical use. There are several examples for the application of H_∞ control in blood glucose regulation [10-11].

When the difference between the nominal model and real patient dynamics is bounded and known this approach becomes highly reliable. However, this requirement is probably the greatest limitation since modeling and model validation is a rather difficult task when working with physiological systems, and guarantees are difficult to give. Furthermore, in case of significant nonlinearity the need to ensure robustness with a linear controller can result in poor disturbance rejection [12].

Linear model predictive control (MPC) is another extensively researched method for the same task and became significantly popular over the last decade for a wide range of physiological applications [13].

The formulation of the control rule can incorporate various constraints, and require manageable computational cost in case of affine constraints and linear model. Including a terminal cost in the cost function of the MPC problem formulation can *increase stability* and include other (e.g. robust) controllers in the control rule. However, linear MPC cannot guarantee global stability.

For both MPC and H_∞ controls, *switching control* can be introduced lessening the effects of nonlinearity, and also reflecting the asymmetric significance of the tracking error of the normoglycemic reference signal [14-15]. To be more specific, hypoglycemia (glucose concentration lower than 3,9 mmol/L) is much more dangerous for the patient than hyperglycemia (higher than 6 mmol/L). Defining different controllers or different glucose concentration regions has proven to be effective and we will continue the efforts in this direction.

The analysis and synthesis of these controllers are significantly more complicated than in the linear case, but the achievable performance is potentially better. Nonlinear control-based exact linearization can transform the system's behavior into a linear one [16-17], without simplification, such as linearization in a given working point (Fig. 2).

The resulting linear model will be valid in a much wider range. However, the dimension of the nonlinear system increases exponentially the complexity of defining the control rule.

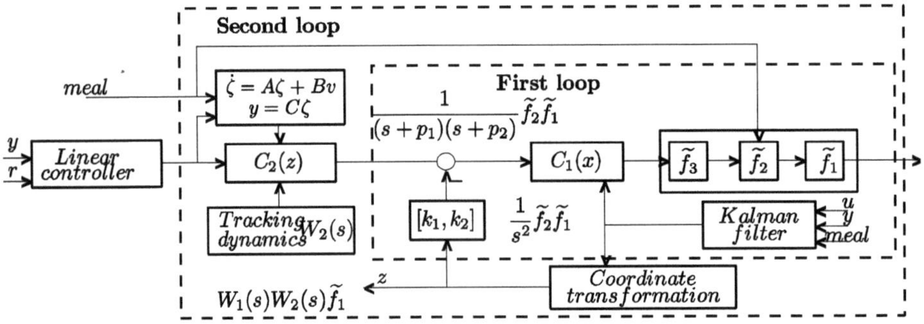

Fig. 2 Structure of nonlinear modeling and control structure realizing asymptotic output tracking control in case of AP problem [17].

Moreover, the method requires the measurement of the state variables, and it can be sensitive to parameter inaccuracies. Although for this problem soft computing techniques are suitable, guarantees are difficult to provide, let it be stability or robustness (constraints can be included, but cannot be strictly enforced).

An effective method that promises the highest disturbance rejection, can handle nonlinearity, hard constraints and certain level of robustness, is *nonlinear MPC* (NMPC) [18]. However, despite these advantages it needs high computation efforts, and is difficult to determine a globally optimal solution.

A suitable choice to compensate the above described problems could be the use of *LPV modeling-based control* [19]. An LPV controller can handle model nonlinearity without approximation, just like exact linearization, but the controller synthesis is significantly easier in comparison even to higher order models. Certain hard constraints can be satisfied as well. To ensure stability and robustness one can define LPV-based robust controllers [20]. The limitations of this approach are the need to measure the time-varying parameters of the LPV formulation and the computational cost for control design.

III. Cancer Modeling and Control: Antiangiogenic Therapy

Cancer diseases are leading causes of death nowadays all around the world. In the EU, the total estimated number of cancer casualties for 2014 was 1.323 million compared to 1.281 million in 2009 [21]. Cancer treatment is an important field in oncology, which may restore regular quality of life or even total recovery for cancer patients. Optimizing treatments would improve efficiency, decrease treatment cost and minimize side effects of cancer therapy. Consequently, the analysis and synthesis of cancer therapies from the control engineering point of view is desirable.

A specific field of cancer treatment is called targeted molecular therapies (TMTs) [22]. These therapies gain more and more importance as they fight specifically against different cancer mechanisms, being more effective and having limited side effects compared to conventional cancer therapies (like chemotherapy, radiotherapy).

Antiangiogenic therapy [23] is a promising TMT arisen in the last decade, which aims to stop tumor angiogenesis (i.e. forming new blood vessels), as without a blood supply tumors cannot grow [24].

However, the corresponding drugs are very expensive and in high doses they may have severe side effects. Protocols for cancer treatment are determined empirically and comprise constant drug dosage, which can be effective in terms of reducing the progression of the disease.

Consequently, from multidisciplinary point of view, the aim is to design a controller which on the one hand is able to minimize the injected dosage (input signal) as far as possible (in order to have less side effects and greater cost-effectiveness) and on the other hand results in appropriately low tumor volume, i.e. stabilizes the state of the patient.

The only existing clinically validated tumor growth model was published in 1999 by Hahnfeldt et al [24]. The Hahnfeldt-model and its simplified form [25] have been used by most researchers working in the field of antiangiogenic control [26]. The tumor volume dynamics is defined by (nonlinear) Gompertzian growth reflecting the empirical fact that the tumor volume has a specific upper limit, and describes the tumor volume reduction due to the endothelial reduction. Different control strategies have been designed on this problem [27-28]; hence, the objective could be the possibility to switch from standardized therapeutic protocols to optimal, individualized therapies under a robust control framework.

IV. Modeling and Control of Control of Anestesia

In general anesthesia consists of three components acting simultaneously on the patient's vital signals (Fig. 3).

i) *Hypnosis* is a general term indicating unconsciousness. The level of hypnosis is related to the infusion of hypnotic drug. Hypnosis is relatively well characterized and sensors to measure it by means of electroencephalogram (EEG) data are currently employed in standard clinical practice [29], while advanced control algorithms and online estimation of variables were applied and investigated [30-31].

ii) *Neuromuscular blockade* ensures that the patient remains paralyzed during surgical procedures and is also a relatively well-characterized process with standard sensors available (EMG-electromyography) [32].

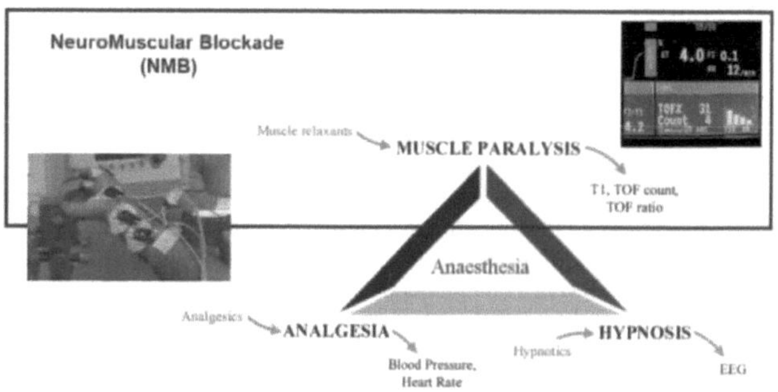

Fig. 3 Control of anesthesia with respect of the neuromuscular blockade closed-loop [32-33].

iii) *Analgesia* represents the loss of pain sensation from an interruption in the nervous system pathway between the sense organ and the brain. Finally, sedation refers to a combined effect of hypnosis and analgesia.

The mathematical interpretation and modeling of these components placed in a control engineering framework (closed-loop computer control of drug-delivery systems and general anesthesia) gives a challenging task that could lead in a decrease of the hospitalization period and minimization of the healthcare costs as well.

Acknowledgment

L. Kovacs is supported by the Janos Bolyai Research Scholarship of the Hungarian Academy of Sciences.

References

1. Zhou K, Doyle JC (1998) Essentials of Robust Control, Prentice Hall.
2. Farkas M (2001) Dynamical Models in Biology. Academic Press.
3. Isidori A (1997) Nonlinear Control Systems I-II, Springer,
4. Mohammadpour J, Scherer CW (2012) Control of Linear Parameter Varying Systems with Applications, Springer.
5. Ljung L (1999) System Identification: Theory for the User, Prentice Hall.
6. Bonzino J (2006) The Biomedical Engineering Handbook, CRC.
7. Wilinska ME, Chassin LJ, Acerini CL, Allen JM, Dunger DB, Hovorka R (2010) Simulation environment to evaluate closed-loop insulin delivery systems in type 1 diabetes, J Diab Sci Techn, 4(1):132-144.
8. Magni L, Raimondo DM, Dalla Man C, De Nicolao G, Kovatchev B, Cobelli C (2009) Model predictive control of glucose concentration in type 1 diabetic patients: An in silico trial, Biomed Sign Proc Contr, 338-346.
9. Palerm CC (2011) Physiologic insulin delivery with insulin feedback: A control systems perspective, Comp Meth Progr Biomed, 102(2):130-137.
10. Colmegna P, Sanchez Pena RS (2014) Analysis of three T1DM simulation models for evaluating robust closed-loop controllers, Comp Meth Progr Biomed, 113(1):371-382.
11. Kovács L, Szalay P (2012) Possibilities and Boundaries of H∞ control in Type 1 Diabetes, Proc. 8th IFAC BMS, Budapest, Hungary, pp 61-66.
12. Szalay P, Eigner Gy, Kovács L (2014) Linear Matrix Inequality-based Robust Controller design for Type-1 Diabetes Model, Proc. 19th IFAC WC, Cape Town, South Africa, pp 9247-9252.
13. Kovatchev BP, Cobelli C, Renard E (2010) Multi-national study of subcutaneous model-predictive closed-loop control in type 1 diabetes: summary of the results, J Diab Sci Techn, 4:1374-1381.
14. Doyle FJ (2012) Zone model predictive control of an artificial pancreas, Proc. 10th WCICA, Beijing, China, pp 8-9.
15. Szalay P, Eigner Gy, Kozlovszky M, Rudas I, Kovács L (2013) The significance of LPV modeling of a widely used T1DM model, Proc. 35th IEEE EMBC, Osaka, Japan, pp 3531-3534.
16. Palumbo P, Pizzichelli G, Panunzi S, Pepe P, De Gaetano A (2011) Tests on a virtual patient for an observer-based, closed-loop control of plasma glycemia, Proc. 10th IEEE CDC-ECC, Orlando, USA, pp 6936-6941.
17. Kovacs L, Szalay P, Benyo B, Chase GJ (2011) Asymptotic output tracking in blood glucose control. A case study, Proc. 50th IEEE CDC-ECC, Orlando, USA, pp 59-64.
18. Zarkogianni K, Vazeou A, Mougiakakou SG, Prountzou A, Nikita KS (2011) An Insulin Infusion Advisory System Based on Autotuning Nonlinear Model-Predictive Control, IEEE J Biomed Eng, 58(9):2467-2477.
19. Kovács L, Benyó B, Bokor J, Benyó Z (2011) Induced L2-norm minimization of glucose-insulin system for Type I diabetic patients, Comp Meth Progr Biomed, 102(2):105-118.
20. Kovács L, Szalay P, Almássy Z, Barkai L (2013) Applicability Results of a Nonlinear Model-Based Robust Blood Glucose Control Algorithm, J Diab Sci Techn, 7(3):708-716.
21. Malvezzi M, Bertuccio P, Levi F, La Vecchia C, Negri E (2014) European cancer mortality predictions for the year 2014, Ann Oncol, 25(8):1650-1656.
22. Gerber DE (2008) Targeted therapies: a new generation of cancer treatments, Am Fam Physician, 77(3):311-319.
23. Pluda JM (1997) Tumor-associated angiogenesis: mechanisms, clinical implications, and therapeutic strategies, Semin Oncol, 24(2):203-218.
24. Hahnfeldt P, Panigrahy D, Folkman J, Hlatky L (1999) Tumor Development under Angiogenic Signaling: A Dynamical Theory of Tumor Growth, Treatment Response, and Pstvascular Dormancy, Cancer Res, 5:4770-4775.
25. Ledzewicz U, Schättler H (2005), A synthesis of optimal controls for a model of tumor growth under angiogenic inhibitors, Proc. 44th IEEE CDC-ECC, Sevilla, Spain, pp 934-939.
26. Ledzewicz U, Schättler H (2009) On an extension of a mathematical model for tumor anti-angiogenesis, Nonlin Anal, 71:2390-2397.
27. Kovács L, Szeles A, Sápi J, Drexler DA, Rudas I, Harmati I, Sápi Z (2014) Model-based Angiogenic Inhibition of Tumor Growth using Modern Robust Control Method, Comp Meth Prog Biomed, 114:98-110.
28. Sápi J, Drexler DA, Harmati I, Sápi Z, Kovács L (2012) Linear state-feedback control synthesis of tumor growth control in antiangiogenic therapy, Proc. 10th IEEE SAMI, Herlany, Slovakia, pp 143-148.
29. Struys M, Versichelen L, Byttebier G, Mortier E, Moerman A, Rolly G (1998) Clinical usefulness of the bispectral index for titrating propofol target effect-site concentration, Anaesth, 53:4-12.
30. Ionescu C, De Keyser R, Claure-Torrico B, De Smet T, Struys M, Normey-Rico J (2008) Robust predictive control strategy applied for Propofol using BIS as a controlled variable during anesthesia, IEEE T Biomed Eng, 55(9):2161-2170.
31. Ionescu C, Hodrea R, De Keyser R (2011) Variable time-delay estimation for anesthesia control during intensive care, IEEE T Biomed Eng, 58(2):363-369.
32. Martins da Silva M, Wigren T, Mendonça T (2012) Nonlinear Identification of a Minimal Neuromuscular Blockade Model in Anesthesia, IEEE T Contr Sys Techn, 20(1):181-188.
33. Sebastiao R, Silva M, Gama J, Mendonca T (2011) Contributions to an advisory system for changes detection in depth of anesthesia signals, LEMEDS Workshop, Bled, Slovenia, pp 1-11.

Author: Levente Kovács
Institute: Obuda University
Street: Becsi ut 96/b.
City: Budapest
Country: Hungary
Email: kovacs.levente@nik.uni-obuda.hu

Real-Time Evaluation of Repetitive Physical Exercise Using Orientation Estimation from Inertial and Magnetic Sensors

Goran Šeketa, Dominik Džaja, Sara Žulj, Luka Celić, Igor Lacković, and Ratko Magjarević

University of Zagreb Faculty of Electrical Engineering and Computing, Unska 3, 10 000 Zagreb, Croatia

Abstract— **Human motion tracking has an important role in a wide variety of applications, including physical exercise. Exercise tracking systems based on the combined use of inertial and magnetic sensors (also called IMU systems) have witnessed a fast increase in popularity in recent years due to their high accuracy and portability. Nonetheless, a complete solution that would guide a user in correctly performing a movement and provide a real-time evaluation of the performed movement is still not available. This paper presents an IMU based system for human motion tracking and its application in real-time evaluation of repetitive physical exercise. The user is provided with a visual demonstration of the correct exercise execution and his own movements. An algorithm is used to compare the movements, thus enabling quantitative and qualitative exercise assessment. However, only simple exercises (that include one limb motion) have been tested with this system, and evaluation of more complex movements shall be explored in the future.**

Keywords—**physical exercise, evaluation, real-time, IMU, inertial and magnetic sensors**

I. Introduction

Accurate tracking of human motion has an important role in a wide range of applications like entertainment, sports, military purposes, robotics, medical applications etc. The choice of technologies for human motion tracking depends significantly on the targeted field in which the obtained data would be used. Considering the equipment and technologies used, systems for motion tracking can roughly be divided into two groups: optical systems and non-optical systems.

Optical systems use a set of cameras and special markers attached to a subject's body to acquire the positions of markers in 3D space. An example is the widely used Vicon system [1]. With the use of optical systems, a highest accuracy in motion tracking can be achieved. The drawbacks however are the system's complexity and high costs. To capture complex movements, a large number of cameras is needed and the setup of such systems is time consuming. Therefore, optical systems are rarely used outside of specialized laboratories. The commercially available, portable, low-cost optical systems (i.e. Microsoft Kinect [2]) are still lagging behind the more expensive systems in terms of the achieved accuracy.

A big variety of non-optical motion tracking systems can be found in the literature: exoskeleton systems [3], e-textil [4], magnetic systems [5] and inertial systems [6,7,8]. Due to high accuracies that can be achieved, mutual combination of the latter two systems is also often used. This combination is popularly called Inertial Measurement Unit (IMU). Some examples of commercial, IMU based, human motion capture systems are the Xsens system [9], Intersense [10] and Trivisio [11]. High prices of such commercial systems often urge researchers to build their own systems for motion based research like in [8, 12-17].

Existing motion tracking systems are mostly used to track rehabilitation progress or aerobic performance during an exercise session [18]. Only few systems deal with strength exercises and none of them provides fully guided exercise tracking with real-time performance evaluation and visual feedback. Recofit system developed by Morris et. al. [8] can successfully track execution of a repetitive exercise through an arm-worn inertial sensor. Nonetheless, this system does not provide guidance how to correctly perform a movement nor a feedback regarding the quality of the movement. Bleser et. al. [19] reported a platform that assists, motivates and supervises elderly people in regular physical exercise. Although some visual and audio feedback is provided, this system also misses the mentioned guidance.

This paper presents a system for human motion tracking and its application for real-time evaluation of a repetitive physical exercise. For the purposes of this work, only one, small low-cost IMU sensor node is used, but more sensor nodes can easily be included in the system for future research. The main purpose of the presented system is to enable a guided exercise execution with quantitative and qualitative real-time evaluation of a performed movement/exercise.

II. System Overview

A. Hardware and Communication

For the assessment of physical exercise motion data, a sensor node is used. The sensor node comprises of four main components: a microcontroller LPC1347 with an implemented Real Time Operating System (FreeRTOS), triaxial inertial and magnetic sensors (accelerometer ADXL345, gyroscope L3G4200D, magnetometer HMC5883L), an RF communication module and a power

Á. Jobbágy (ed.), *First European Biomedical Engineering Conference for Young Investigators*,
IFMBE Proceedings 50, DOI: 10.1007/978-981-287-573-0_3

supply. The sensor node is powered by a rechargeable Li-ion battery attached to the node. This makes the sensor node fully autonomous in movement (no need for power or data cables).

The microcontroller reads measurements taken by sensors with a frequency of 55 Hz and forwards them wirelessly to a PC through an Access Point. In order to optimize power consumption and achieve better performance, a customized communication protocol based on TCP/IP is used for data transfer [20].

B. Orientation Estimation

The sensor node gyroscope measures angular velocities in three axes, which can be integrated over time to compute the sensor's orientation. However, the integration of gyroscope measurement errors leads to an accumulating error in the calculated orientation and therefore the gyroscope alone cannot provide an absolute measurement of orientation. On the other side, accelerometer and magnetometer measure Earth's gravitational and magnetic fields that may be used to obtain an absolute measure of orientation. Nonetheless, they are likely to be subject to high levels of noise; for example, accelerations due to motion corrupt measured direction of gravity. In order to resolve these issues related to the use of individual sensors for orientation estimation, an algorithm (filter) can be used for the computation of a single estimate of orientation through the optimal fusion of gyroscope, accelerometer and magnetometer measurements.

Kalman filter is the most commonly used algorithm for orientation estimation problems in commercial motion tracking devices (e.g.. Xsens [9], Intersense [10]) due to its accuracy and effectiveness. The implementation of the Kalman filter imposes however a large computational load, making it an not optimal choice for small low-power microcontrollers. The Madgwick filter [21] is an alternative algorithm that achieves levels of accuracy matching that of the Kalman filter, but with much lower computational load and the ability to operate at small sampling rates. This algorithm uses a quaternion representation, allowing accelerometer and magnetometer data to be used in an analytically derived and optimized gradient descent algorithm to compute the direction of the gyroscope measurement error as a quaternion derivative [21]. These improvements significantly reduce the hardware and computational power necessary to implement the Madgwick filter compared to the Kalman filter and thus make the Madgwick filter a better solution for applications where battery life is of big importance. For all this reasons, the Madgwick filter was implemented as an optimal solution for the sensor node orientation estimation.

As already mentioned, Madgwick filter outputs the estimated orientations in the unit quaternion representation. Quaternions, that form a four-dimensional vector space, are proven very useful in representing rotations due to several advantages, above the other representations. Although less intuitive than Euler angles, they are simpler to compose and avoid the problem of gimbal lock. Compared to rotation matrices on the other hand, they are more numerically stable and may be more computationally efficient.

C. Sensor Calibration

Accelerometers, gyroscopes and magnetometers that are used to provide necessary measurements for orientation estimation belong to the MEMS sensors family. They provide a digital output value proportional to the measured physical quantity. The use of an estimation algorithm requires that this value is converted to a suitable engineering unit. These units are obtained by accounting for a calibrated bias and gain in the sensor output. Due to the mechanical properties of MEMS devices, the characteristics of an individual sensor cannot be guaranteed during manufacture and may be altered after manufacture when soldered. Consequently, no two sensors may be guaranteed to be the same and each should be uniquely calibrated. Therefore, a set of measurements was collected from every sensor at a known orientation (for accelerometer and magnetometer) and angular velocity (gyroscope) in order to calculate the sensor gain and bias.

Additionally, magnetometer measurements may be corrupted by magnetic interferences fixed to the sensor frame (hard-iron distortions) or by ferromagnetic materials around the sensor that change the density of Earth's magnetic field locally (soft-iron distortions). Magnetometer measurements subject to hard and soft-iron distortions lie on the surface of an ellipsoid which can be accurately modelled by twelve parameters. The calibration process consists of fitting the twelve model parameters to a set of measurements using Merayo technique [22]. The method tries to find the best 3D ellipsoid that fits the measurements and returns the parameters of this ellipsoid. When these parameters are known, the magnetometer measurements can simply be transformed from the surface of the ellipsoid to the surface of a sphere centered at the origin. This algorithm must however operate upon a set of data which describes as completely as possible the 3D space and may fail with too poor data.

D. Motion Tracking and Virtual Scene

In order to track human motion with the previously described technology, human body must first be represented by a model. For the purposes of this work, a slightly altered version of Hanavan's model is used [23]. The human body is thereby modelled as a pure kinematic chain consisting only of rigid body parts with well-defined ball-and-socket joints. When a sensor node is attached to the user's body with an elastic band, it can be assumed that each orientation estimation derived from the sensor node measurements corresponds to a respective body segment orientation. The position of a particular body part is then simply derived from the estimated orientation and the known body part length with the use of forward kinematics.

From this body model, two 3D characters were created using *MakeHuman* software [24] and placed in a virtual scene with *Unity 3D* game-engine. Hence, the virtual scene consists of two characters: a virtual trainer and user's avatar. The virtual scene is included in the user's application and serves for visualization of the performed motion [25]. Virtual trainer serves as a substitute for a real-life trainer and visually guides the user to perform an exercise correctly. The user's avatar on the other hand shows the real-time movement of the user tracked with the sensor node.

To match the actual body part position to the virtual scene character, several computations are required. Before the start of each exercise, the user is asked to stand still in a neutral position (standing with arms beside the body) for which the orientations of body segments are *a priori* known. In this position, the initial orientation is taken. Every estimated orientation during a movement is then multiplied by the complex conjugate of this initial orientation. The result of multiplication is a quaternion that describes the rotation from initial orientation to the current orientation. The quaternion that represented orientation relative to Earth's global reference coordinate system is thereby converted to an orientation relative to some arbitrary initial coordinate system. Additionally, the resultant quaternion must be inverted from a right-handed coordinate system (coordinate system attached to the sensor node) to a left coordinate system to match the virtual scene coordinate system. Finally, initial body part positions of the virtual character are multiplied by quaternion rotations computed in the previous step to perform the wanted motion of the virtual character.

III. REAL-TIME EXERCISE EVALUATION

For the purpose of quantitative and qualitative exercise evaluation, 10 simple exercises (e.g. lateral and front arm raise, shoulder dumbbell press etc.) performed at three different speeds (slow, medium, and fast) were recorded and stored in a database. Every record represents all orientations obtained from the sensor node during one representative movement. To achieve the wanted repetition number in a repetitive exercise, these recoded movements can be repeated arbitrary number of times. Only exercises that are traceable with one sensor node were recorded.

The recorded movement is presented to the user via the virtual trainer character. User should try to follow the movements performed by the trainer. A real-time visual feedback is provided to the user of his own actions through the other virtual character – user's avatar.

In order to evaluate an exercise, movements of the virtual trainer are compared to the movements of the user's avatar. The comparison is made by calculating the dot (inner) product of orientation quaternions of a body segment in virtual trainer and user's avatar. Taking the dot product of two quaternions gives a scalar value proportional to the difference between the two orientations represented by these quaternions. At the beginning of a movement, an initial score is assigned to the user. With every orientation estimation obtained from the sensor node measurements, the quaternion dot product is calculated, scaled and subtracted from the score. The more the user's body segment orientation differs from the correspondent recorded orientation, the more points are subtracted from the score. Finally, a decision is made by the end of the movement by comparing the final score to empirically set thresholds in order to validate whether the performed movement can be acknowledged as a valid exercise repetition. Additionally, at the end of the exercise, based on the ratio of valid and total number of repetitions, an algorithm decides whether the exercise in general was successful.

The virtual scene consisting of a virtual trainer and user's avatar during one exercise execution is shown in Figure 1. The above described algorithm is used to evaluate the exercise and provide a real-time feedback to the user about the success of the performed movement.

IV. DISCUSSION AND CONCLUSION

This paper describes a system for real-time evaluation of repetitive physical exercise. For this purpose, a sensor node consisting of inertial and magnetic sensors is used. Characters in a virtual scene guide the user in performing the wanted movements and provide an immediate visual feedback to the user.

Initial studies have shown that the evaluation algorithm successfully differentiates user's movements that follow the guidance of the virtual trainer from those that are significantly different. The evaluation algorithm threshold value can thereby be used to set up the tolerance level for how much one allows a user to deviate from the referent, recorded movement.

For our future work, we plan to include more sensor nodes in the system and evaluate complex exercises that involve simultaneous movements of various body parts. Also, a performance evaluation will be performed in order to test the system performance compared to some commercial motion tracking devices.

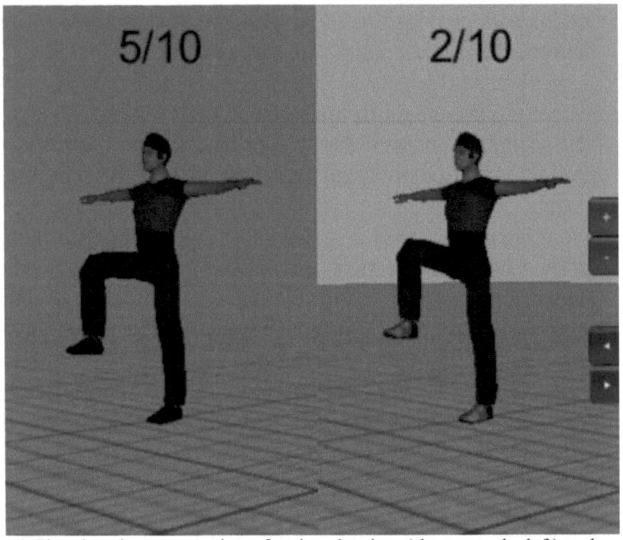

Fig. 1 The virtual scene consists of a virtual trainer (shown on the left) and user's avatar (on the right). Numbers above virtual trainer's character (5/10) indicate the number of so far demonstrated repetitions (5) and the total number of repetitions that shall be performed. The numbers above user's avatar (2/10) show the number of successfully performed repetitions in the total number of repetitions (10).

Acknowledgment

The research leading to these results has partially received funding from the Central Finance and Contracting Agency of the Croatian Ministry of Science, Education and Sports under agreement n° RC.2.2.08-0010

Conflict of Interest

The authors declare that they have no conflict of interest

References

1. Vicon [Online] Available: www.vicon.com, Accessed: 2015-02-09
2. Microsoft Kinect [Onlin Available: http://www.microsoft.com/en-us/kinectforwindows/default.aspx, Accessed: 2015-02-09
3. ReWalk [Online] Available: http://www.rewalk.com, Accessed: 2015-02-09
4. Lim, C.K.,Chen, I.M. et. al. (2010). A low cost wearable wireless sensing system for upper limb home rehabilitation. Proc. IEEE Conf. Robot. Autom. Mechatronics., 2010, pp. 1–8.
5. Polehemus [Online] 2015. Available: http://polhemus.com, Accessed: 2015-02-09
6. Silva, B. De, Natarajan, A., Motani, M., et. al. (2008). A real-time exercise feedback utility with body sensor networks. 5th International Summer School and Symposium on Medical Devices and Biosensors, 2008. pp. 49–52.
7. Haapalainen, E., Laurinen, P., Roning, J., & Kinnunen, H. (2008). Estimation of Exercise Energy Expenditure Using a Wrist-Worn Accelerometer: A Linear Mixed Model Approach with Fixed-Effect Variable Selection. Seventh International Conference on Machine Learning and Applications, 2008. pp. 796–801
8. Morris, D., Saponas, T. S., Guillory, A., Kelner, I. (2014). RecoFit. In Proceedings of the 32nd annual ACM conference on Human factors in computing systems - CHI '14. New York, New York, USA, 2014. pp. 3225–3234
9. Xsense [Online] Available: www.xsens.com, Accessed: 2015-02-09
10. Intersense [Online] Available: www.intersense.com, Accessed: 2015-02-09
11. Trivisio [Online] Available:www.trivisio.com, Accessed: 2015-02-09
12. Lee, W. W., Yen, S.-C., Tay, E. B. A.,et. al. (2014). A smartphone-centric system for the range of motion assessment in stroke patients. IEEE Journal of Biomedical and Health Informatics, 18(6), pp. 1839–47
13. Buonocunto, P., & Marinoni, M. (2014). Tracking limbs motion using a wireless network of inertial measurement units. Proceedings of the 9th IEEE International Symposium on Industrial Embedded Systems (SIES 2014), pp. 66–76.
14. Lin, Z., Zecca, M., Sessa, S., et. al. (2011). Development of the wireless ultra-miniaturized inertial measurement unit WB-4: Preliminary performance evaluation. Proceedings of the Annual International Conference of the IEEE Engineering in Medicine and Biology Society, EMBS, 6927–6930.
15. Brigante, C. M. N., Abbate, N., Basile, A., et. al. (2011). Towards miniaturization of a MEMS-based wearable motion capture system. IEEE Transactions on Industrial Electronics, 58(8), 3234–3241.
16. MacEdo, P., Afonso, J. A., Rocha, L. A., Simoes, R. (2014). A telerehabilitation system based on wireless motion capture sensors. In PhyCS 2014 - Proceedings of the International Conference on Physiological Computing Systems, pp. 55–62
17. Brückner, H.-P., Krüger, B., & Blume, H. (2014). Reliable orientation estimation for mobile motion capturing in medical rehabilitation sessions based on inertial measurement units. Microelectronics Journal, 45(12), pp. 1603–1611.
18. Patel, S., Park, H., Bonato, P., Chan, L., & Rodgers, M. (2012). A review of wearable sensors and systems with application in rehabilitation. Journal of NeuroEngineering and Rehabilitation, 9(1), 21.
19. Bleser, G., Steffen, D., Weber, M., et al. (2013). A personalized exercise trainer for the elderly. Journal of Ambient Intelligence and Smart Environments, 5(6), pp. 547–562.
20. Celic, L., Varga, M., Pozaic, T., et al. (2013). WBAN for Physical Activity Monitoring in Health Care and Wellness, IFMBE Proc. vol. 39, World Congress on Medical Physics and Biomedical Engineering, Beijing, China, 2013, pp 2228-2231.
21. Madgwick, S. O. H, Harrison, A. J. W, Woidyanathan, R (2011). Estimation of IMU and MARG orientation using a gradient descent algorithm. 2011 IEEE International Conference on Rehabilitation Robotics Rehab Week Zürich ETH, Switzerland, July 2011.
22. Merayo, P., Brauer, P., Primdahl, F., Petersen, J.R., Nielsen, O.V (2000). Scalar calibration of vector magnetometers. Measurement Science and Technology, Vol. 11, No 2., February 2000.
23. Hanavan E.P.A. A Mathematical Model of the Human Body. 1964.
24. MakeHumanand its Purpose [Online] 2014. Available: www.makehuman.org/doc/node/makehuman_and_its_purpose.html, Accessed: 2015-02-09
25. Zulj, S.,Seketa, G., Dzaja, D., et. al (2014). Virtual Reality System for Assisted Exercising Using WBAN. IFMBE Proc. vol 45, 6th European Conference of the International Federation for Medical and Biological Engineering, Dubrovnik, Croatia, 2014. pp 719-723.

Author: Goran Seketa
Institute: University of Zagreb, Faculty of Electrical Engineering and Computing
Street: Unska 3
City: Zagreb
Country: Croatia
Email:goran.seketa@fer.hr

Cylindrical Cell-Based Refractometers to Analyse Biomedical Liquids

D. Merkulovs[1], Y. Dekhtyar[1], O. Vilitis[2], P. Shipkovs[3], and V. Merkulova[4]

[1] Riga Technical University, Riga, Latvia
[2] Institute of Solid State Physics, University of Latvia, Riga, Latvia
[3] Institute of Physical Energetic, Latvian Academy of Science, Riga, Latvia
[4] ELMI Ltd, Riga, Latvia

Abstract— **Compact device of high sensitivity for measurement of the refractive indices of both stationary and flowing liquids has been developed. This device can be used to analyse a variety of biomedical liquids: urine, serum protein. The refractive index (RI) is determined by measuring the deviation of a laser beam passing through a cylindrical cell containing the test liquid. In order to significantly improve the resolution and stability of RI measurements, the repeated reflections and refractions of the light beam travelling through the cylindrical cell are employed.**

Keywords — **refractive index, refractometer, optical cell, cuvette, laser.**

I. Introduction

Conventionally the refractometers are in use to identify the concentration of sugar in the blood and urine, protein in the urine; analyse blood serum, brain and joint fluids; urine and intraocular liquid density, etc.

The refractive index (RI) of a liquid carries important information about its density and component concentration. This is important for fundamental research, chemical analysis and medical diagnostics.

The aim of the present article is to exhibit the method that has several times enhanced resolution and stability of RI measurements for transparent and low absorbent liquids. The technique is applicable also for unclear, absorbent liquids, turbid colloidal suspensions and liquids with gas or solid particle inclusions. To relate the RI to the concentration of the liquid component, the calibration should be provided.

Typically the device [1, 2] is equipped with the laser beam that is optically connected to a linear image sensor through a thin-walled cylindrical cell containing the analysed liquid.

The direction of the beam travelling via the cell is detected by the sensor and is stipulated by the liquid RI. The presented device increases the sensitivity of RI measurement, specified as the derivation *dx/d(RI)* where **a** - position of the beam on the coordinate sensitive light detector, has been increased multiple times by recurring reflection and refraction of the beam on its way through the cylindrical boundary between the material of the cell and the liquid, as described in [2, 3]. The proposed approach allows the beam to cross the liquid four times or more.

II. Principles of Functioning of the Optical Cell

A schematic cross section of the cylindrical cell (cuvette) showing a simplified route of the beam in the measuring system is exhibited in Fig.1. The refractometers measuring system consists of a laser diode, a cylindrical thin-walled cell with its cross section perpendicular to the axis **O** of the cylinder and a linear image sensor. The cell is filled with either immobile or flowing liquid. The position **a** of the beam is identified using a linear CMOS image sensor.

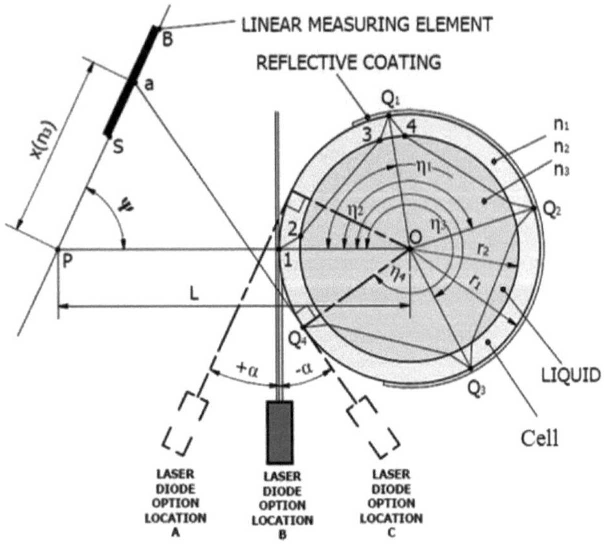

Fig. 1. Schematic cross section of the cylindrical cell is illustrating a simplified path of the laser beam in the measuring system.

The laser beam axis is lined up with the cell's outer wall tangent and is perpendicular to the axis of the cylinder. The laser beam after refraction at point **1** crosses the medium of the cell's wall and arrives at point **2** on the boundary between the material of the cell's inner wall and the liquid.

Á. Jobbágy (ed.), *First European Biomedical Engineering Conference for Young Investigators*,
IFMBE Proceedings 50, DOI: 10.1007/978-981-287-573-0_4

The experiments evidenced that in the vicinity of the critical angle the beams intensity of light is the highest [2].

For this reason, to illustrate the trajectory of the coherent light beam in the cylindrical cell, Fig.1 shows only the path of rays that are close to the critical angle. After being refracted at the boundary point 2, light rays travel through the test liquid and, having crossed it, fall upon the inner wall of the cylinder at point 3, where they are refracted again and reach the point Q_1 through the medium of the cell's wall.

Because the outside surface of the cylinder is coated with a reflective film the rays falling on this unit area of the boundary surface are reflected and intersect the cell's wall and the liquid several times in a similar way.

The analytical calculation of the RI of liquids contained in the system described above is given in [6], where applying the laws of light refraction and reflection and using simple trigonometric formulae, the central angle η_m (see Fig.1 for the case when m=4) was calculated as:

$$\eta_m = 2m[(\pi/2 - \arcsin(k/n_3) + \arcsin(k/n_2) - \mathrm{asin}(1/n_2) + \alpha] \quad \text{rad}, \quad (1)$$

where $k = r_1 / r_2$ is the ratio of the outer and inner radii of the cylindrical cell; n_2 and n_3 are the refractive indices of the material of the cell and the liquid, respectively; α - central angle of the laser impact position in the tangential line on the lateral surface of the cell. The angle α must be taken into account in Eq.(1) for adjusting the laser beam entering the sensitive surface of the linear optical element, to cover the whole measuring range of the refractometer. If the laser beam enters the sensitive area of the linear optical element, it is necessary to provide the deviation of the angle in a clockwise direction, the sign is positive; when the deviation of the angle is contraclockwise, this sign is negative. See Fig.1.

III. Results of the Experimental Tests of the Measuring Device

The measuring device was used to estimate the advantages of the developed method for detection of the position of the image had the following optical and geometrical parameters: m=4; n_2=1.5151; r_1=5.5mm; r_2=4.5mm; L=5+5.5mm; ψ=90°, α=68°.

An 5 mW, λ=632.8 nm miniature laser diode is used as the light source. A *Hamamatsu* CMOS monochromatic linear 1024 pixel image sensor S9226 with the pixel width 0.0078 mm is used.

The position of the image was detected using the position of the first minimum of the waveform light intensity distribution [3-6] over the image sensor.

The solutions have been prepared by using a precision hydrometer (for calibration of ethanol aqueous solutions) and precision weighing instrument (for calibration of NaCl and sucrose aqueous solutions), at standard temperature of 20°C (concentration - %weight/vol.). Refractometer has been placed in a specially made thermostat with the temperature setting of ±0.1°C and maintain the desired temperature with accuracy ±0.05°C. For the temperature measurements, a platinum thermal sensor (resolution ±0.02°C) was in use. The mathematical computation of the temperature-compensated ($c_{\%TC}$) concentration (% weight/vol.) of a given liquid sample is based upon a polynomial calibration equation (obtained as shown below). In order to illustrate the proposed computations, an example for thermo-compensated measuring device was provided.

Calculation of the thermo-compensated volume concentration of a binary liquid sample was carried as follows.

- Splitting of the measurement range of sample concentration into smaller. The range from 0% to 20% weight/vol.
- Preparation and arranging of the measured data p_s (Table 1) by ascending percentages of concentration. Recording of the measured concentration of the reference sample $c_{\%R}$ value p_s set to the measured sample temperatures t_f 15°C, 20°C and 25°C.
- Using the p_s values (Table 1) obtained at the sample temperature of 15°C, to perform a regression analysis. Similarly, using the appropriate values measured at the sample temperature of 20°C and 25°C the following calibration equations were obtained.

Table 1 Measured n_s values arranged by ascending percentages of the reference sample concentration $c_{\%R}$ and by measured sample temperatures t_f

Concentration, $c_{\%R}$	Temperature, t_f	Measured p_S
0 %	15°C	230
	20°C	197
	25°C	164
5 %	15°C	397
	20°C	368
	25°C	339
10 %	15°C	578
	20°C	552
	25°C	526
15 %	15°C	747
	20°C	724
	25°C	701
20 %	15°C	895
	20°C	874
	25°C	854

• The volume percent ethanol concentration ($c_{\%}$) depending on the p-values according to the calibration equation was approximated:

$$C_{\%15} = -8.44003 + 0.04251 \cdot p - 2.97694 \cdot 10^{-5} \cdot p^2 + 1.98727 \cdot 10^{-8} \cdot p^3, \quad (t=15°C), (2)$$

$$C_{\%20} = -6.87204 + 0.03931 \cdot p - 2.60827 \cdot 10^{-5} \cdot p^2 + 1.86354 \cdot 10^{-8} \cdot p^3, \quad (t=20°C), (3)$$

$$C_{\%25} = -5.4247 + 0.03624 \cdot p - 2.19761 \cdot 10^{-5} \cdot p^2 + 1.68678 \cdot 10^{-8} \cdot p^3, \quad (t=25°C), (4)$$

The squared correlation coefficient corresponding to Eqs. (2), (3) , (4) is $R^2=1$, $R^2=1$, $R^2=0.9999$ accordingly.

Refractometer is designed as a multi-purpose device, it was necessary to provide the calibration process by taking into account the 3rd order polynomials. This is done in order to have a possibility to use the refractometer for other solutions in the future and also automatically include in the calibration process the effect of temperature influences of all constructive components of this device. When calibrating the refractometer to concentrations of alcohol the input of elements p^2 and p^3 in the equations were not enough, and the result of this was some linear relationship, which we have used to define the resolution.

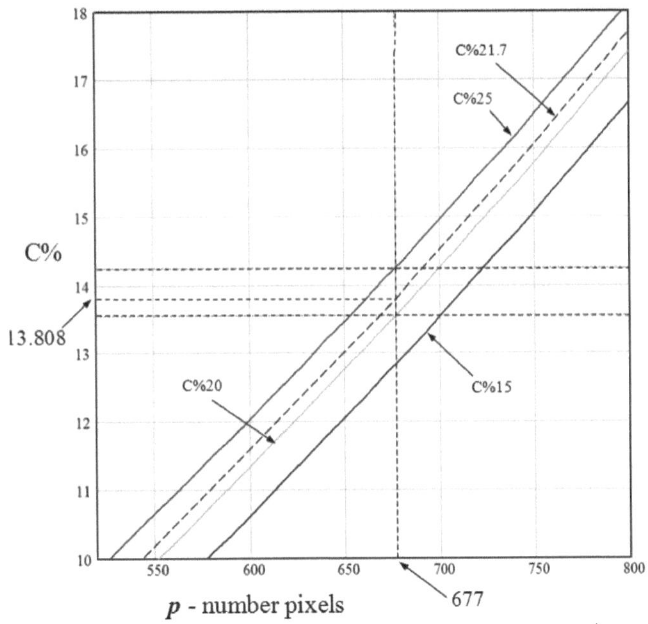

Fig. 2. The calculated thermo-compensated weight concentration $C_{\%}$ for a given ethanol-water mixture sample at the actual measured sample temperature t_m.

Calculation of the thermo-compensated volume concentration $C_{\%TC}$.

For $+15°C < t_m < 20°C$:

$$C_{\%TC} = C_{\%15} + [(C_{\%15} - C_{\%20})(20 - t_m)]/\Delta t, \quad (5)$$

where $\Delta t = 20 - 15 = 5$.

For $+20°C < t_m < 25°C$:

$$C_{\%TC} = C_{\%20} + [(C_{\%20} - C_{\%25})(20 - t_m)]/\Delta t, \quad (6)$$

where $\Delta t = 25 - 20 = 5$.

Doing exemplary calculation of the thermo-compensated volume concentration $C_{\%TC}$ of a given ethanol-water mixture sample:

a) For the actual sample temperature t_m and concentration p (expressed in notional units p) measured and fixed using the developed measuring device.

For the chosen sample the values t_m = 21.7°C and p=677 are measured and recorded.

b) Using Eq.(3) and Eq.(4) and assuming p=677, the following volume percentages are obtained:

$C_{\%20} = 13.569\%$ and $C_{\%25} = 14.271\%$

c) Substituting the above $C_{\%}$ values, for t_m=21.7°C the thermo-compensated liquid measured concentration is calculated by the Eq.(6), as a result, will have: $C_{\%TC} = 13{,}808$.

The microcontroller of the sensor unit performs the calibration and recording of measured data as well as processes the data of the previous example, and records the final results.

For the refractometer for ethanol aqueous solutions, accordingly, at t=+15°C, n_3=1.33264, and at t=25°C, n_3=1.33158. [7] Measurements show that the first minimum of the optical intensity distribution changes its position from pixel p=230 at t_1=+15°C to pixel p=164 at t_2=+25°C. In accordance with the given parameters of the optical system, the resolution of the measuring device $\delta = \delta_n / \delta_p$ (where $\delta_n = |n_1 - n_2|$ is the difference in refractive indices, $\delta_p = |p_1 - p_2|$ the difference in detected positions) before mathematical processing of the data is about $\delta = 1.6 \cdot 10^{-5}$ measurable RI units per pixel.

Analogue, the measured resolution δ per pixel for RI and concentrations of ethanol, NaCl and sucrose aqueous solutions for refractometers. (See Table 2).

Table 2. The measured resolution δ per pixel for RI and concentrations of ethanol, NaCl and sucrose aqueous solutions for refractometers

Ethanol, range, % weight/vol	0-20
$\delta_{ethanol}$, RI units	1.6×10^{-5}
$\delta_{ethanol}$, % weight/vol	0.03
NaCl, range, % weight/vol	0-9
δ_{NaCl}, % weight/vol	0.011
Sucrose, range, % weight/vol	0-10
$\delta_{sucrose}$, % weight/vol	0.013

CONCLUSIONS

(1) The new configuration of the device for high accuracy measurement of the refractive index of liquids has been developed

(2) The laser beam is directed to cross the measured liquid four or more times. The novel approach to process the probe light beam front projected to the coordinate sensitive detector has been reached. The procedure increases stability and sensitivity of the RI measurements.

(3) Empirical results and calculations demonstrate that the developed optical system provides the resolution of $1.6x10^{-5}$ measurable RI units even if the distance between the cylindrical cell and the linear measuring element does not exceed 5 mm.

(4) The applicability of CCR to identify concentrations of ethanol, NaCl and sucrose were tested. The corresponding resolutions of 0.03%, 0.011%, 0.013% weight/vol.

REFERENCES

1. Vilitis O. and Merkulov D. (2004) Optical cell for measuring refractive index and concentration of liquids. Latv.J.Phys.Technol.Sci. 4 58-66
2. Vilitis O., Merkulov D. and Kozlov V. (2003) Method and refractometer for measuring refractive index of liquids. Patent LV 13294 B
3. Vilitis O. and Merkulov D. (2006) Method for detecting optical image of the light beam in refractometer. Patent LV 13598 B
4. Vilitis O., Merkulov D. and Shipkovs P. (2007) Method and sensor for measuring concentration of liquids. Patent LV 13728 B
5. Vilitis O., Shipkovs P. and Merkulov D. (2008) Determination of refractive index of liquids using a cylindrical cuvette. Latv.J.Phys.Technol.Sci. 3 50-62
6. Vilitis O., Shipkovs P. and Merkulov D. (2009) Determining the refractive index of liquids using a cylindrical cuvette. Measurement Science and Technology 8pp DOI: 10.10088/0957-0233/20/11/117001
7. Harvey A. H., Gallagher J. S. and Levelt Sengers J. M. H. 1998 Revised formulation for the refractive index of water and steam as a function of wavelength, temperature and density J. Phys. Chem. Ref. Data 27 773

Author: Dmitrijs Merkulovs
Institute: Riga Technical University
Street: Ezermalas 6
City: Riga
Country: Latvia
Email: dmitrijs_merkulovs@yahoo.co.uk

Development of the Mobile PoC Graphene-Based Biosensing Device Using Electrochemical Impedance Spectroscopy (EIS)

Daniel Matias[1], Łukasz Przeniosło[1,2], Tomasz Miłosławski[1], Marek Jaskuła[1], Przemysław Makiewicz[1], Marcin Biegun[1], Krzysztof Penkala[1], Ewa Mijowska[3], Mirosława El Fray[4], and Jacek Podolski[5]

[1] West Pomeranian University of Technology, Department of Systems, Signals and Electronics Engineering, Szczecin, Poland
[2] West Pomeranian University of Technology, Faculty of Electrical Engineering, Department of Systems, Signals and Electronics Engineering, Biomedical Engineering Student Research Group "AKSON",Szczecin, Poland
[3] West Pomeranian University of Technology, Institute of Chemical and Environment Engineering, Department of Nanotechnology, Szczecin, Poland
[4] West Pomeranian University of Technology, Department of Biomaterials and Microbiological Technologies, Szczecin, Poland
[5] NZOZ "Meditest. Diagnostyka Medyczna" Jacek Podolski, Szczecin, Poland

***Abstract*— In the paper the results of research on a multifunctional graphene-based biosensor are presented.**

Project of a mobile device is described for Point-of-Care (PoC) diagnostic tests based on Electrochemical Impedance Spectroscopy (EIS) and Bioelectrical Impedance (BI) technique, using integrated impedance scanner AD5933 (Analog Devices). Design of a biosensing electrode, a control circuit based on XMEGA microprocessor, and results of preliminary experiments and simulations are also presented.

***Keywords*— Biosensing, graphene, biosensing electrode, EIS, Electrochemical Impedance Spectroscopy, BI, Bioelectrical Impedance, BIA, Bioelectrical Impedance Analysis, impedance scanner, microprocessor system, PoC, SoC, simulation**

I. INTRODUCTION

Sensitive, selective, rapid, efficient, and low cost analysis of different biomolecules and microorganisms is a key factor in clinical practice when performing different diagnostic tests. It is also essential for good results of patient treatment. Hence, there is a growing demand for decentralized laboratory methodologies which can be implemented in a clinic, in doctor's office, emergency room or in the field for analysis of such targets as DNA, RNA, proteins, antibodies, bacteria, viruses, small compounds etc. Lab-on-a-Chip (LoC) platforms and miniaturized Point-of-Care (PoC) devices based on biosensors fulfill these demands and are foreseen to revolutionize future medical diagnostics. Because of excellent electrical, mechanical and optical properties, graphene has recently found to be highly attractive in biosensing applications, and potentially may thrust new perspectives into the field of miniaturized medical diagnostic devices. Graphene-based biosensors are advantageous in terms of, for example, large detection area, possibilities of new sensing mechanisms, ease of effective functionalization, immobilization of other particles on its surface, and – finally – good biocompatibility.

The main objective of the "Multifunctional graphene-based biosensor for medical diagnosis" project, conducted in years 2013-2015 within the framework of the GRAF-TECH Programme, is to develop a biosensor for effective electrochemical detection of specific DNA microbial targets in biological samples and blood glucose monitoring. This technology will allow fabrication of low cost sensing components and devices for PoC diagnosis. More universal laboratory version of the graphene-based biosensing system will be also developed.

The project contributes to technology progress in the field of graphene-based biosensors, giving a strong thrust to the development of clinically approved miniaturized micro-nano-electronic devices for PoC diagnosis. It is also presumed that clinical evaluation of performance of developed graphene biosensors, which is an important aspect of this project, will attract more attention from biomedical devices industry and future investment allowing more rapid technology development.

In the study current state is presented of our work on biosensor electrodes as well as electronic systems for reading the signal and for control of measurement procedures. The mobile PoC version of the developed device is described.

II. ELECTROCHEMICAL BIOSENSING – BI/EIS TECHNOLOGY

One of technologies applied in development of the multifunctional graphene-based biosensor is Electrochemical Impedance Spectroscopy (EIS). Within this methodology, Bioelectrical Impedance (or Bioimpedance – BI) measurements are performed. In general, in medicine BI technology is used for diagnostic purposes, including biosensing, and the so-called Bioelectrical Impedance Analysis (BIA), which is a noninvasive method of body composition analysis [1-3]. The BI method is increasingly popular also in sports medicine, aesthetics medicine and dietetics. Several

Á. Jobbágy (ed.), *First European Biomedical Engineering Conference for Young Investigators*, IFMBE Proceedings 50, DOI: 10.1007/978-981-287-573-0_5 manufacturers offer specialized electronic equipment for professional body composition measurements based on bioimpedance analysis [3].

A. BIOSENSING ELECTRODE CONCEPT

The project of a mobile PoC biosensing device involves the use of two-, and three-electrode setup for performing the measurements. Sensor should be sensitive and selective for effective electrochemical detection of DNA fragments of microorganisms (bacteria, viruses) and other biomolecules in biological material [4]. Figure 1 shows the concept of the 1st generation bio-sensing element for preliminary experiments to use with different types of sensing probes.

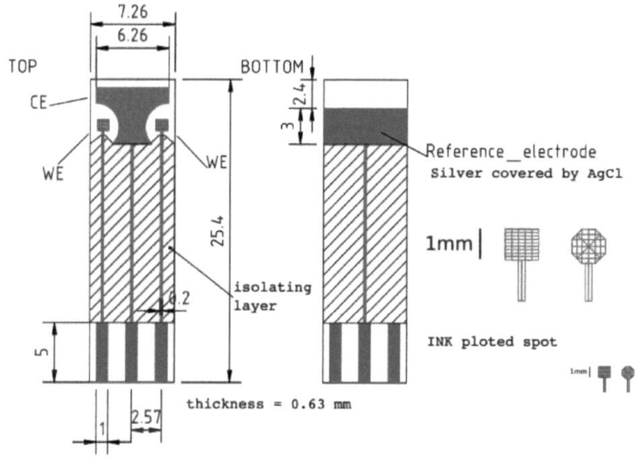

Fig 1. Concept of the 1st generation bio-sensing element

It consists of three electrodes: 1 – WE (working electrode), 2 – RE (reference electrode), 3 – CE (counter electrode). The material for the substrate is specially modified polymer. The aim of the modification is to activate the surface that allows printing with specially prepared chitosan-graphene inks. These inks are composed of three main components: chitosan, graphene functionalized with heteroatoms (N, B) or metal nanoparticles (Pd, Pt, Au, Fe, Ag, Ni) and probes that are complementary with target DNA. Doping graphene with heteroatoms and metal nanoparticles increase electron transfer speed and biosensor sensitivity. The main component of the sensor is working electrode. This is an active region where the process of hybridization occurs. On the top of the biosensor are placed two WE electrodes. One is functionalized with probes, the other not. This is in order to get the result at the same time from functionalized and not functionalized electrodes.

B. CONTROL CIRCUIT

Taking under consideration all of the requirements, we decided to use for mobile PoC graphene-based biosensing device the ATXMEGA128A1U microcontroller produced by Atmel (AVR architecture). This module covers all needs of the application, leaving some "free space" for hardware and software expansions which are likely to take place when using the device for research purposes. Also its capacities are much better than standard AVR and PIC microcontrollers for the same price. On Figure 2 the schematic diagram of the microprocessor BI-measurement system is shown.

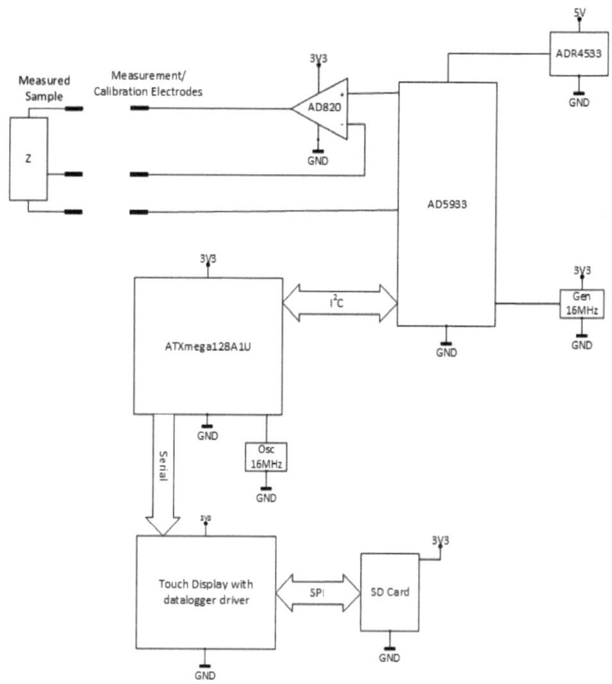

Fig 2. Block diagram of the microprocessor-based BI-measurement system (explanations in the text)

For development work in a stage of design, two evaluation boards were used: EVAL-AD5933EBZ (Analog Devices) with the integrated impedance scanner AD5933 and a popular development board with the ATXMEGA128A1U microcontroller (Atmel). Then the own evaluation board was designed and built (Figure 3), in order to conduct optimization of algorithms and characteristics for measurement systems dedicated to specific applications of the BI-EIS technology (e.g. biosensing, body composition analysis, analysis of blood parameters etc.).

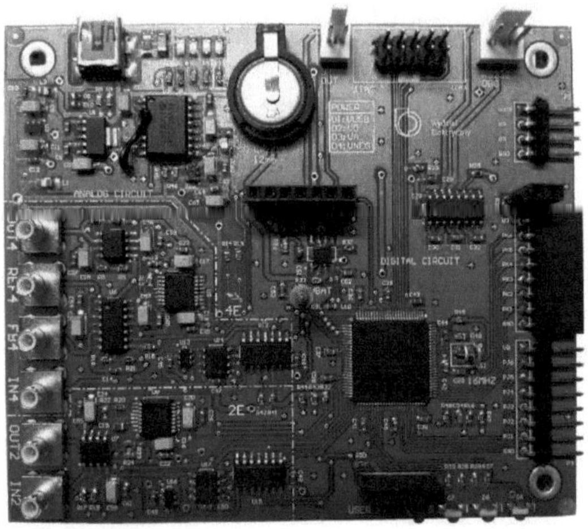

Fig 3. Bioimpedance measurement platform – own evaluation board

In biosensing application, in order to ensure constant conditions (in particular temperature range, so critical in the process of hybridization and amplification of the DNA), it was necessary to design a special housing for the mobile PoC version of the device, with the thermostatic chamber. Figure 4 shows 3D model of the device enclosure.

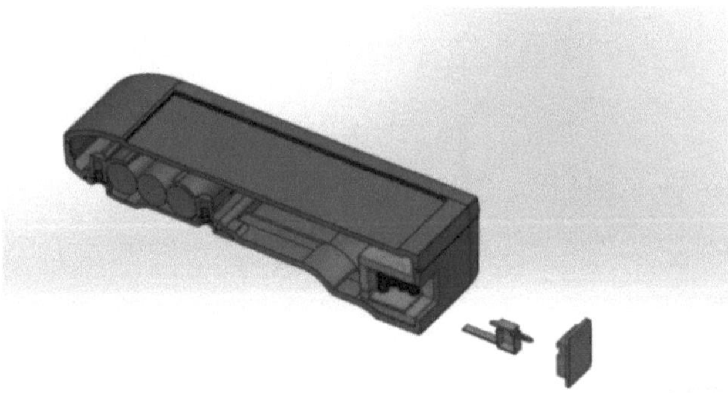

Fig 4. 3D model of the PoC version enclosure

III. PRELIMINARY EXPERIMENTS AND SIMULATIONS

The results of impedance measurements for electrical model of the tissue (Figure 5), performed with the use of integrated circuit AD5933, were compared with the results of simulation carried out in the PSpice program for this model. Results of this comparison are shown on Figure 6 and Figure 7 [5]. Both impedance frequency characteristics showed satisfactory similarity.

Recently new measurements for the same model were performed with the use of the Autolab system (Metrohm, Netherlands) which served as a reference platform in our studies on electrochemical biosensing technology. Again, good agreement between results was obtained (Figure 8).

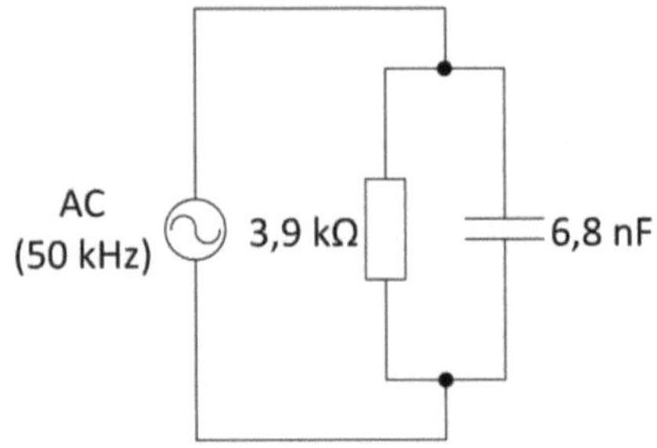

Fig 5. Electrical model of the human tissue

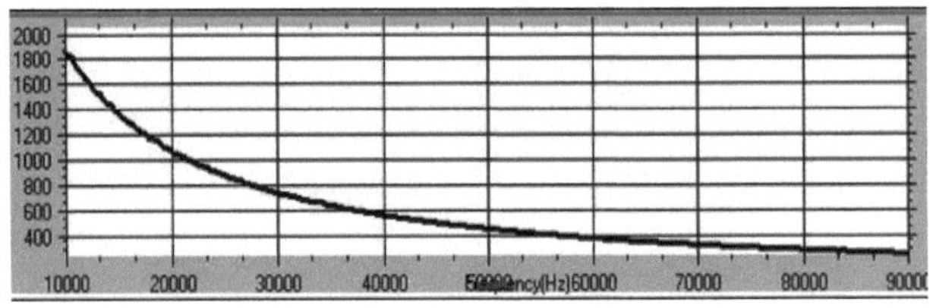

Fig 6. Measurements performed with the AD5933 integrated circuit

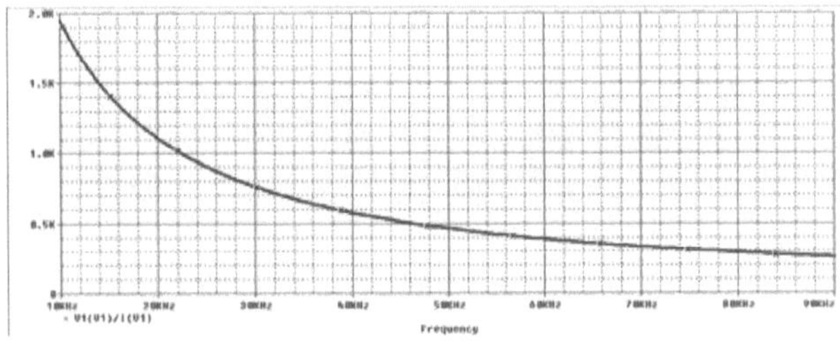

Fig 7. Results of simulation in the PSpice program

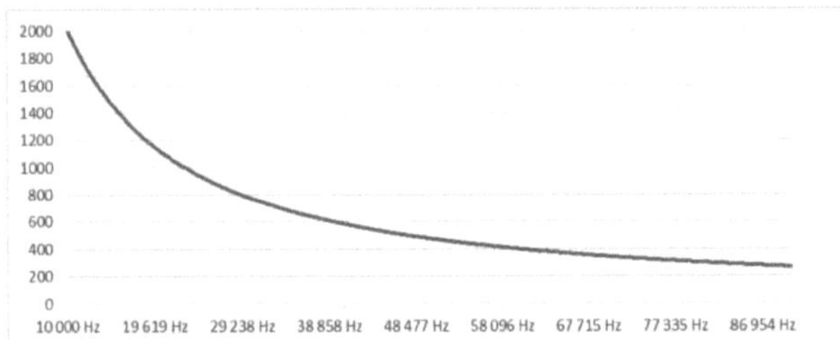

Fig 8. Measurements performed with the Autolab system

We also obtained similar compatibility of results in comparative measurements for physiological solutions with the use of AD5933, and two commercial BIA systems: Bodycomp-MF (Akern, Italy) and Quantum II (JBL, USA). Maximum differences of the values of impedance did not exceed a few percent (Table 1).

Tab.1. Impedance measurements for physiological solutions

Device	EVAL-AD5933EBZ	Quantum II	BodyComp-MF
Solution/frequency	**50 kHz**		
NaCl 0,002 M	1100 Ω	1092 Ω	904 Ω
NaCl 0,01 M	153 Ω	150 Ω	145 Ω

IV. CONCLUSIONS

The results of comparative impedance measurements fully justify the use of AD5933 module in BIA research. System-On-a-Chip (SoC), implemented in the layout, is a full-featured impedance spectroscopy measuring device.

Research tasks for further work, in which it is planned to use the results of current studies, include:

- optimization of the design of bio-sensing electrode,
- optimization of graphene-chitosan ink (concentration, the quantitative ratio of chitosan and graphene),
- optimization of DNA probes (selectivity, concentration),
- optimization of testing frequencies (selecting the best frequency ranges).

Thanks to innovative solutions, it will be possible to achieve commercialization effects for the results of presented research.

ACKNOWLEDGMENT

This project is financially supported by the National Centre for Research and Development within the framework of the GRAF-TECH Programme, grant No. GRAF-TECH/NCBR /08/06/2013.

REFERENCES

1. Kyle U.G. et al.: Bioelectrical Impedance Analysis, part I: Review of Principles and Methods. Elsevier Ltd, 2004
2. Lewitt A., Mądro E., Krupienicz A.: Podstawy teoretyczne i zastosowania analizy impedancji bioelektrycznej (BIA). Via Medica,Warszawa, 2007
3. Lewandowski D., Biedka A., Borkowska K., Penkala K.: Testy funkcjonalne dwóch wybranych urządzeń do analizy impedancji bioelektrycznej (BIA). Inżynieria Biomedyczna - Acta Bio-Optica et Informatica Medica, vol. 16, No. 2, 2010, pp. 83-87
4. Pumera M.: Graphene in biosensing, Materialstoday, vol. 14, no. 7-8, 2011
5. Przeniosło Ł., Walków M., Krzeszewska S., Pisarek S., Biedka A., Jaskuła M., Matias D., Penkala K.: Integrated impedance scanner in selected biomeasurement applications - control circuit. Krajowa Konferencja Studentów i Młodych Pracowników Nauki, Unieście, Poland, May 23, 2013, Zeszyty Naukowe Wydziału Elektroniki i Informatyki Politechniki Koszalińskiej, vol. V, pp. 63-69, Koszalin 2013, ISSN 1897-7421

Corresponding author:

Author: Przemysław Makiewicz
Institute: Department of Systems, Signals and Electronics Engineering, Faculty of Electrical Engineering, West Pomeranian University of Technology, Szczecin, Poland
Street: Sikorskiego 37
City: 70-313 Szczecin
Country: Poland
Email: makiewicz@zut.edu.pl

Six-Axis Strain Gauge Force Sensor for Robot-Assisted Movement Therapy

Márk Ottó Bauer[1], Zsolt Hodosán[1], Mihály Jurák[2], and András Tóth[1]

[1] Department on Manufacturing Science and Engineering BME, Budapest, Hungary
[2] Department of Applied Mechanics BME, Budapest, Hungary

Abstract - **This paper discusses the development of a 6 axis strain gauge force-torque sensor for the REHAROB robotic physiotherapy system. Based on literature review and the study of the former sensor of TARA Electronics Ltd. the transducer was designed and prototyped. Signal processing electronics was also designed and developed. Finally, for calibration purposes a test environment was built and the elements of the calibration matrix were calculated from dedicated series of measurments.**

Keywords -**multi axis, force, torque, sensor, strain gauge, calibration, matrix**

I. INTRODUCTION

Accelerating development of bio- and medical robotics calls for more and more smart sensors, among others force and torque sensors. In most of the industrial cases it is sufficient to measure the loading force-torque vector at end-of-arm tooling along one or two spatial axes, but the spreading force control techniques presents an increasing need for advanced, multi-axis force-torque measurement. In industrial robotics it is almost the only solution when a 6 axis force-torque sensor is placed between the flange and the tool in order to measure the loading of the tool. Two custom-made force–torque sensors were used in the REHAROB physiotherapy robot system just the same way. The sensors were developed by TARA Electronics Ltd. for reasons like small size, easy mechanical integration with a custom made manual tool changer and integration of the outer-loop force control algorithm into the signal processing DSP.

In this paper the development of a new 6 axis force-torque measuring sensor with improved characteristics is discussed. The development was justified by the following reasons: recently introduced active therapy in REHAROB required a sensor with same shape and interface but increased load capability, and overload protection range.

II. LITERATURE REVIEW

A. Analysis of the damaged sensor

We have analysed one of six-axis force-torque sensor of TARA Electronics Ltd. used previously in the REHAROB physiotherapy robot system and was damaged due to overloading during testing. We have identified the outputs of the strain gauges with using the general resistant measuring method. Four beams connect an inner ring with an outer ring (Fig. 1). Each beam is mounted with 6 strain gauges, which form full bridges with their pairs, thus 12 half-bridges are wired to the output connector. Based on the review of the technical literature it can be stated that such differential measuring usually features good signal noise ratio between the sensor and the signal processing unit even in case of long extension cords like in the case of REHAROB.

After encoding the electronics the next step was the analysis of the mechanical structure. Firstly the sensor geometry was digitalised then its CAD model was built (Fig. 1). The main geometrical features of the sensor were designed for standard machining (like turning, milling). Furthermore the sensor's inner ring has a central hole through which the leading of electricity, air, or mechanical power is possible. The lightweight structure of the sensor implies that rigid mechanical interfaces are required both at the robot side and at the tool side.

B. Structural design of transducers

Richard A. Meyer and co-inventors describe in their patent [2] a special sensor which is able to measure axle load of vehicles while the shaft is rotating. In their sensor two discs were connected with axial rods on the circumference of the discs. Another transducer structure is the cross bridged structure patented by Tetsuro Sakano [4]. In Sakano's solution there are also rods that connect two discs like in [3]. The rods have special T-shaped heads distributed evenly along the circumference of the disc. The structure of Junquing Ma and Aiguo Song [1] is identical with the structure of TARA Electronics Ltd. except minor differences. From manufacturing and assembly point of view this structure can be considered as ideal.

III. DESIGNING AND MANUFACTURING THE SENSOR BODY

While we followed the literature and standard engineering practice in the design of the transducer a number of innovative solutions have also been proposed for

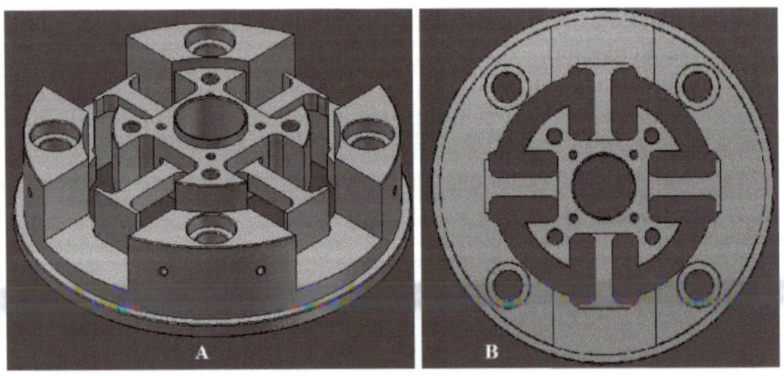

Fig 1 3D CAD model of the damaged sensor

Á. Jobbágy (ed.), *First European Biomedical Engineering Conference for Young Investigators*,
IFMBE Proceedings 50, DOI: 10.1007/978-981-287-573-0_6

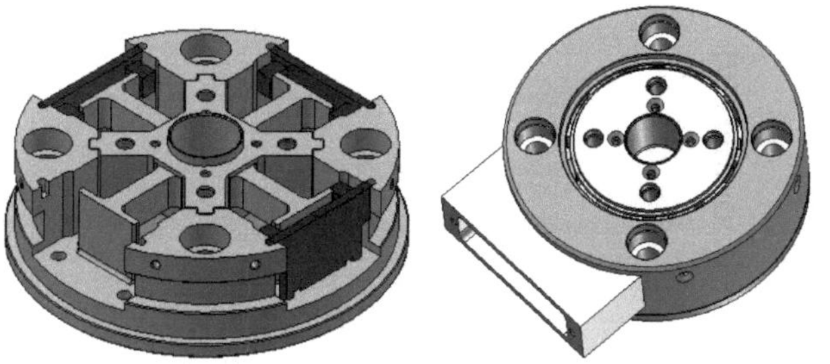

Fig 2 Interior with built-in printed circuit boards and the exterior of the new transducer

mechanical overload protection and shaping for gluing and cabling the strain gauges. Mechanical overload protection has been achieved by stressing the Aluminium deformable for 50-100 [MPa] at maximum while preventing any further axial and/or radial deformation by resting the deformable element on another rigid surface of the transducer. Sophisticated 3D wire EDM technology was the key enabler of this innovation that effectively protects the sensor from frequent mechanical shocks like robot collisions, spasm of the patient, nonlinear loading in singular configuration.

Ideal place for internal electronics was also found. Fig. 2 shows the interior of the transducer with built-in printed circuit boards (in blue). The upper and lower rings' functions, shown on the right-side model, are overload-inhibition and insulation against external dust and vapour (the strain gauge resistors are sensitive to meteoric humidity).

It can be asserted that the new design of the sensor in terms of both reliability and aesthetics is an improved design.

A. Verification of the mechanical geometry

Parallel to designing the geometry, we performed finite element tension and strain analysis by Inventor and ANSYS software platforms. An example of the results is shown on Fig. 3. Critical load is the torque vector of 1500 [Ncm] parallel to the Y or Z direction. The maximum equivalent tension are 250 [MPa], this provides the 2[-] safety factor. The X-axis 2500 [Ncm] torsional torque provides a 2.1 [-] safety factor. Loaded by planar force, the maximum

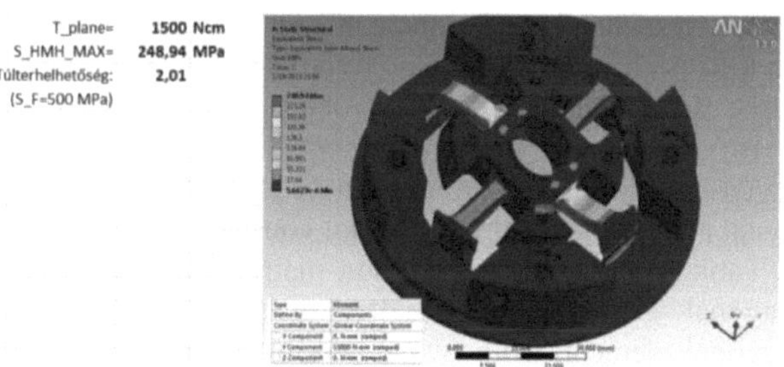

Fig 3 Loaded by torque along axis Y

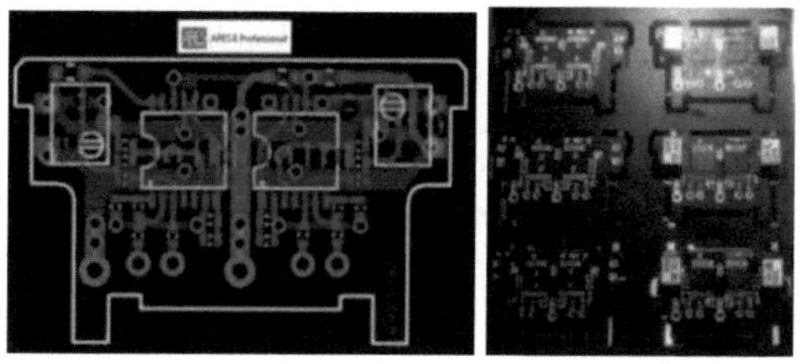

Fig 4 PCB drawing and production of the amplifier

tensions is coupled, if line of action of the force between the two ribs run at 45 degrees, the prescribed force was 200[N], with a 3.7 [-] value of safety. Axial (X-axis) force is the highest safety factor given: 6.9[-] at 300 [N]. Mechanical design requirements with using high solidity easy to work CERTAL (AL7075T6) type aluminium have been fully attained during the iterations.

IV. SIGNAL PROCESSING ELECTRONICS

A. Selecting the strain gauge

The new column elements have bigger areas for the strain gauges what gave the opportunity to apply strain gauges – type KMT-LIAS-06-1.5/350-6EL: straight grid oriented, 1.5mm nominal grid length, 350 ohm, grid covered strain gauge [5] - with longer active grid length.

B. Attachment of the strain gauge to the load cell elements

Gluing (glue selection, sanding the surface for roughness varying between 12-25[μm], glue application, curing, strain gauge placement with marking under microscope) is of fundamental quality issues of the transducer. One displaced strain gauge can only be corrected in the bridge externally with offset tuning. We have followed the best practices but due to space limits no details can be disclosed.

The wiring was made in the way to provide both half bridges with the same supply power wire branch. In Figure 4 the wiring drawing can be seen.

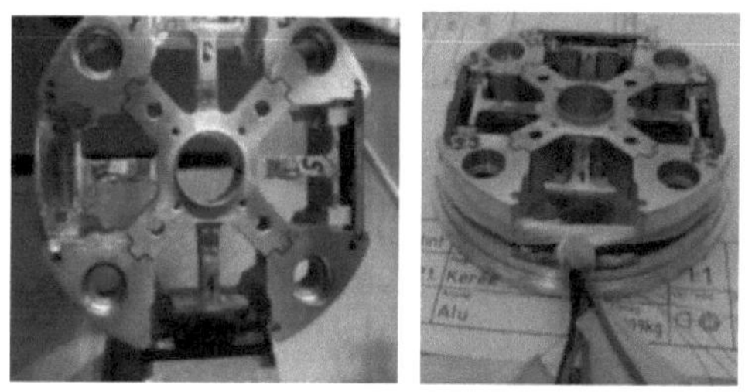

Fig 5 Fully wired transducer with signal processing electronics inserted into three slots (right)

C. Signal amplifier

The selected operational amplifier is a smaller sized, MCP664 chip. This operational amplifier provides rail-to-rail type output (Fig. 4). In Figure 5 fully wired and completed strain gauge load cells are shown. Raw sensor signals are being amplified by 40dB (divided amplification), from 5[V] to ±10[V]. A big advantage is the improved signal to noise ratio, moreover the sensor itself has a usable output level.

V. Calibration of the Load Cell

A. The Process of Calibration

The purpose of the calibration is *to find the accurate* relation *between the external forces and the resultant voltages* measured on the strain gauges of the load cell. That can be closely approximated by a first order linear matrix transformation.

Takeshi Ohsato and *Yusuke Hirabayashi* presented the detailed steps of the mathematical operations for obtaining the calibration matrix [3]. Their theory was followed in this paper by similar steps.

The linear relation between the forces and the voltages can be determined by applying known loads in accurately determined positions and measuring the resultant output voltages. We can write equation (1) that defines the problem:

$$\bar{F} = \bar{\bar{T}} \cdot \bar{q} \qquad (1)$$

where:

$\bar{F}$ – the *known force vector*

$\bar{\bar{T}}$ – the *unknown calibration matrix* to be determined

$\bar{q}$ – the *recorded voltage vector* as a response to the force vector

Matrix $\bar{\bar{T}}$ in this form could not be determined with direct measurements, therefore left multiply the equation with $\bar{\bar{T}}^{-1}$we obtain:

$$\bar{q} = \bar{\bar{B}} \times \bar{F} \qquad (2)$$

Where $\bar{\bar{B}}$ denotes the inverse transformation matrix $\bar{\bar{T}}^{-1}$.

According to *Takeshi et al* the columns of matrix $\bar{\bar{B}}$ can be determined in by having only one component other than 0 in the **F** vector – thus applying pure force and torque loads aligned with the axes of the sensor. Pure loads were generated by the well known mechanical principle of superposition property (Fig. 6)

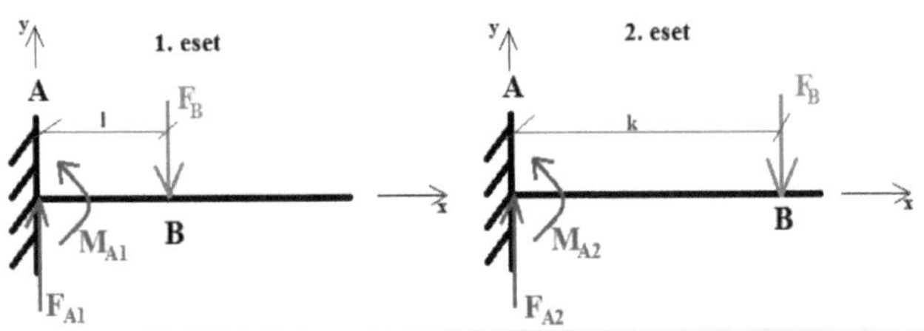

Fig. 6 Applying the same loads at two different positions to the calibration bars.

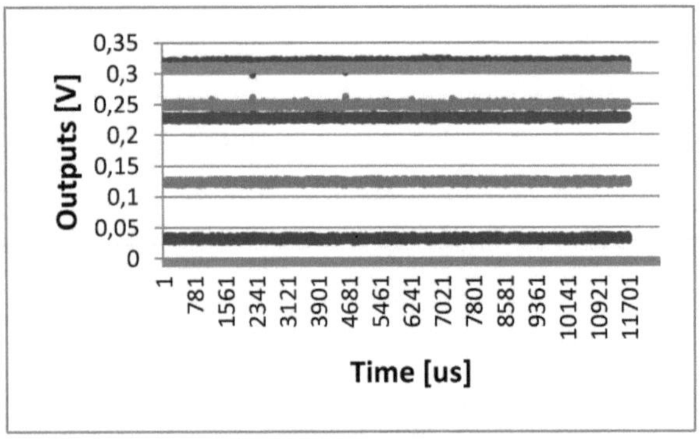

Fig 7 Output voltage levels of the damaged sensor

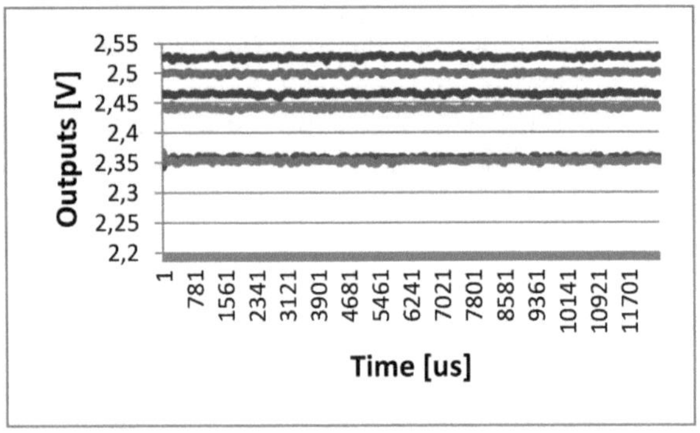

Fig 8 Output voltage levels of the new sensor

If we apply a known F_B force to the loading bar at different distances, the resultant reaction force remains the same, but the torque changes:

$$F_{A1} = F_B \text{ and } M_{A1} = F_B \cdot l \qquad (3)$$

$$F_{A2} = F_B \text{ and } M_{A2} = F_B \cdot k \qquad (4)$$

All columns of the 6x6 transformation matrix can be determined in three different planes. The redundant measurements provide possibility for either double checking the calculated values, or reducing the effect of the noises measurement – calculating the average of the two corresponding values.

B. Validation of the sensors

Figure 7 and Figure 8 show the output voltage signals of the damaged and the new sensors respectively. Standard deviation of the output signals at Fig. 7 is 2.08[mV] while peak-to-peak value of the blue trendline (Fig. 9) is 8.4[mV]. Same parameters for the new sensor are: 1.67[mV] and 2.8[mV] (red trendline). The new sensor has superior signal-noise ratio even if the positive effect of the integrated signal processing electronics is not considered.

Table 1 shows the calibration matrix. Most of the non-diagonal elements are smaller than the corresponding diagonal elements with two orders of magnitude but there are three force related and one torque related elements where the coefficient is only one order of magnitude. This

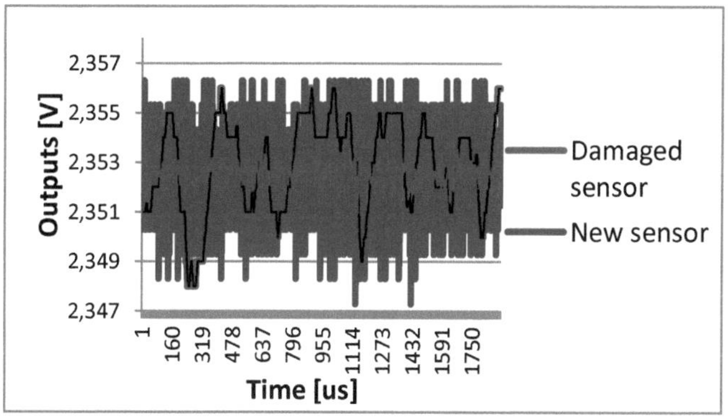

Fig 9 Output voltage levels of the new sensor

implies that the sensor performs much more accurately (-1-4%) in torque measurement than in force measurement. Fig. 10 shows both the linearity, and the cross sensitivity of the sensor for torque measurement.

Table 1 Absolute Transformation matrix

Fx	Fy	Fz	Mx	My	Mz
1.4029	-0.0878	-0.1147	-0.1233	-0.0027	-0.1503
0.0564	*1.7939*	0.0411	-0.0043	0.0037	-0.0262
-0.0173	0.1634	*1.0950*	0.0826	-0.0135	0.0844
0.0020	-0.0061	-0.0322	*0.0202*	-0.0005	-0.0030
0.0043	0.0011	-0.0016	0.0002	*0.0236*	-0.0010
0.0308	0.0011	-0.0034	-0.0028	0.0001	*0.0180*

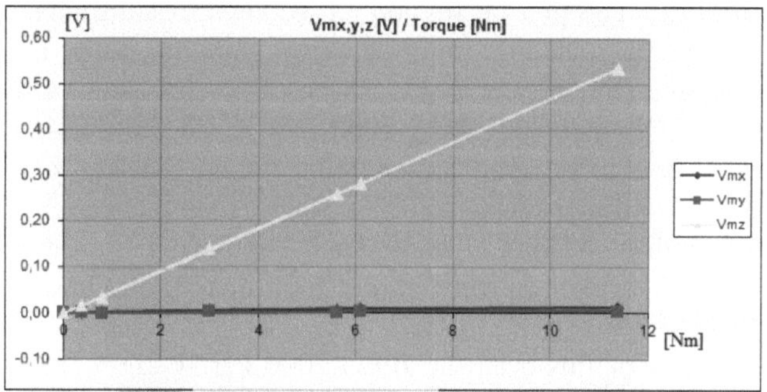

M [Nm]	x	Name	Vmx	Vmy	Vmz
0	0	ZERO	0,00	0,00	**0,00**
0,397	1	Fz m=-2.532kg X=16mm	0,0021	0,0002	**0,0169**
3,006	2	Fz m=-2.532kg X=121mm	0,0051	0,0027	**0,1407**
5,614	3	Fz m=-2.532kg X=226mm	0,0054	0,0022	**0,2587**
0,806	4	Fz m=-5.135kg X=16mm	0,0021	-0,0014	**0,0340**
6,095	5	Fz m=-5.135kg X=121mm	0,0095	0,0037	**0,2827**
11,385		Fz m=-5.135kg X=226mm	0,0130	0,0048	**0,5346**

Fig. 10 Result of torque measurements on axis XZ.

The inferiority of force measurement is demonstrated by Table 2. We have assessed the accuracy of force measurement for the 'Y' axis. It can be observed that by using the calibration matrix of Table 1 the accuracy of the force sensor falls to as weak as to 29%.

We have already identified a number of imprecisions in the production technology such as pairing of and placement of strain gauges, glue selection and curing, cabling and the missing second stage 500x amplifier for a further improved signal-noise ratio.

Table 2 Assessment of accuracy for F_y

Sensor value [N]	Real value [N]	Difference [N]	Deviation [%]
23.92667	24.839	0.912	4
26.26567	24.839	-1.427	-6
21.53297	24.839	3.306	13
49.34361	50.374	1.031	2
40.72612	50.374	9.648	19
35.81513	50.374	14.559	29

VI. Conclusion

In this paper we presented the design, development and calibration of a strain gauge six-axis force and torque sensor for the REHAROB therapeutic robotic system. Despite the inaccuracies described in section V the sensor has been functioning since September 2014. It has worked so far 280 hours over 230 therapeutic sessions. During these months no failure has occurred, the sensor works flawlessly up to this day. Based on the experience gained in design and technology of strain gauge force sensors building of a second improved sensor is in progress.

Acknowledgement

This work was supported by the National Innovation Office, Hungary, under the grant COSMOSYS Nr. TÉT_08-SG-2010-0002.

The publication of the work reported herein has been supported by ETDB at BME.

Conflict of Interest

The authors declare that they have no conflict of interest.

References

1. Junqing Ma, Aiguo Song: Fast Estimation of Strains for Cross-Beams Six-Axis Force/Torque Sensors by Mechanical Modeling. Jiangsu Key Lab of Remote Measurement and Control, School of Instrument Science and Engineering, Southeast University, Nanjing 210096, China, 2013, http://www.mdpi.com/1424-8220/13/5/6669/htm
2. Richard A. Meyer, Alan J. Kempainen, Dougles J. Olson: Multi-axis load cell body, Patent number: US 6769312 B2, (2004), http://www.google.com/patents/US6769312
3. Takeshi Ohsato, Yusuke Hirabayashi: Six-axis force sensor. Patent number: US6823744 B2 (2004), http://www.google.com/patents/US6823744
4. Tetsuro Sakano: Six-axis force sensor. Patent number: US 20060213287 A1, (2006), http://www.google.com/patents/US20060213287
5. Official website of Kaliber Kft (http://kaliberkft.hu)

Author: András Tóth
Institute: Department on Manufacturing Science and Engineering, BME
Street: Műegyetem rkp. 3.
City: Budapest
Country: Hungary
Email: toth@manuf.bme.hu

3D Coding of Volumetric Medical Data Sets

László Tóth

Department of Networked Systems and Services, Multimedia Networks and Services Laboratory
Budapest University of Technology and Economics, Hungary
tothl@hit.bme.hu

Abstract— **Advancements in digital radiology have led to a significant increase of the sample bit-depth and resolution of data sets, causing accordingly grow in size. Both efficient storage and efficient transmission of large medical data sets request efficient compression techniques. In this paper, we investigate the state-of-the-art volumetric medical data compression techniques. We present our web-based interactive test system for storing and visualising 3D medical images, and testing and comparing several compression methods.**

Keywords— **DICOM,JPEG2000,3D Image Coding**

I. INTRODUCTION

The DICOM (Digital Imaging and Communications in Medicine) standard generally is used for the exchange of images and related information. Nowadays, all medical imaging devices (also known as Modality), such as CT, MRI, supports the DICOM standard [1].

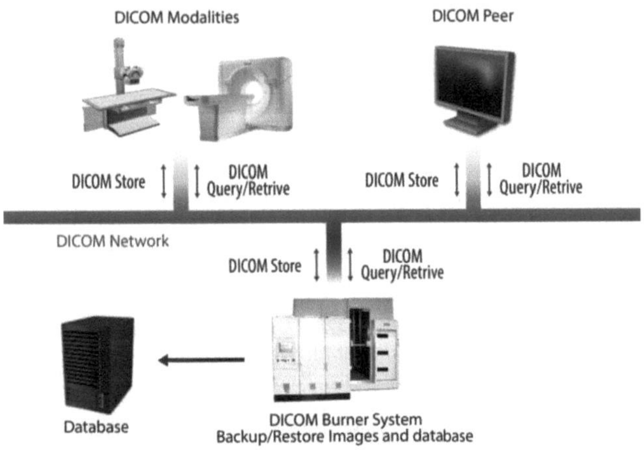

Fig. 1: DICOM Network

The scope of medical imaging is wide, from a digital image of a bone X-ray (a single frame), to a set of tomographic slices through all of the body. Projection X-ray images and reconstructed tomographic slices are grayscale, but typically require encoding with a resolution beyond 8 bits.

Digital medical imaging devices generate large amounts of volumetric data sets. Advancements in digital radiology have led to a significant increase of the sample bit-depth and resolution of data sets, causing accordingly grow in size.

DICOM provided a set of standards that allow for interoperability and compatibility in a multi-vendor eco-system. DICOM technology provides interface between imaging devices and a network, and it makes the communication robust and transparent(Figure 1).

In this paper we investigate the state-of-the-art compression techniques of 3D medical data.

II. THE JPEG 2000 TECHNOLOGY IN MEDICAL DATA COMPRESSION

The JPEG 2000 standard defines a new image-coding scheme using wavelet-analysis based compression techniques [3]. The present version 3.0 adopted existing image compression standards from the JPEG working group. Because promising results of wavelet-based compression methods DICOM adopted JPEG 2000 Part 1, so the standard is able to offer efficient compression, storage and transmission of two-dimensional medical images. Additionally, JPEG 2000 with embedded block coder by optimized truncation (EBCOT) technology delivers excellent quality and bit-rate scalability [4].

In spite of this even the JPEG 2000 Part 1 2D methodology is still considered state-of-the-art image compression technology. In practice, often simple schemes are employed in lossless of medical data. For instance, only incorporating run-length coding is defined in DICOM.

While in everyday use it is tolerable transient inconvenience of having to download a new software (or a new codec) version to view a picture or video, such untrustworthy operation is absolutely unacceptable in the practice of medicine.

DICOM'S one main disadvantage is, that it allows a very limited set of compression methods that can be used both on the network and on offline interchange media[7].

Á. Jobbágy (ed.), *First European Biomedical Engineering Conference for Young Investigators*,
IFMBE Proceedings 50, DOI: 10.1007/978-981-287-573-0_7

III. Implementation and Test System

Aiming to investigate JPEG2000 compression techniques, we have implemented a test system based on JPEG2000 technologies. In common applications these technologies is not widely used.

The JPEG 2000 codec even in FFMPEG is still experimental [1]. (The j2k codec, both encoder and decoder are not lossless nor bitexact with reference jpeg2000 implementations, which explains why they are experimental). For further investigation we had to build an own test system to work with j2k techniques in medical imaging.

We implemented an OpenJPEG based test system for export medical data from DICOM and compression.

All major functionalities, like 2D preview from slices, volume rendered 3D preview, compression method selection, parameter setting, statistics form result are easily accessible from a simple menu.

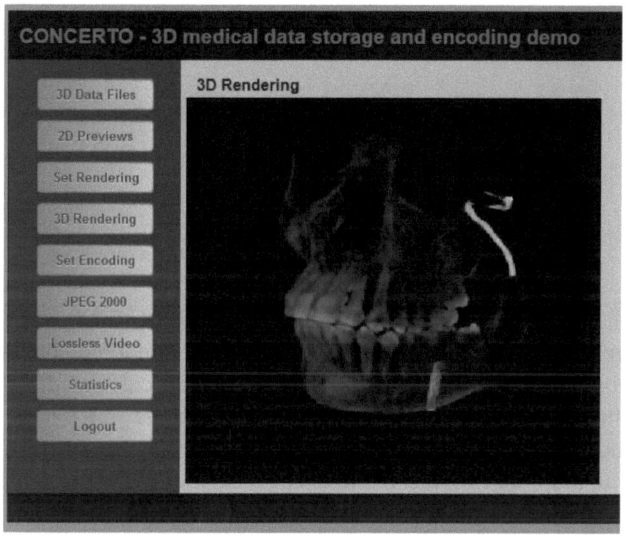

Fig. 2: Web interface of the test system

Many scanning devices, such as CT and MR, result in slices through an object, each 2D slice is presented as a grey scale image. Each pixel in the image corresponds to some characteristic at that point in space, for example X-ray absorbtion in CT scans or protein density in MR.

The 3D medical data storage and encoding test-system, has a web-based user interface, and a database interface for 3D medial data files, where input (original 3D medical data) files can be selected, 2D preview montage can be generated, parameters for directory-based and JPEG2000 encoding can be set, volume rendered image can be generated, statistics about the test results can be viewed. The interface has a simple menu-system, from where each important service avaiable (fig 2).

[1] 2015.02.10

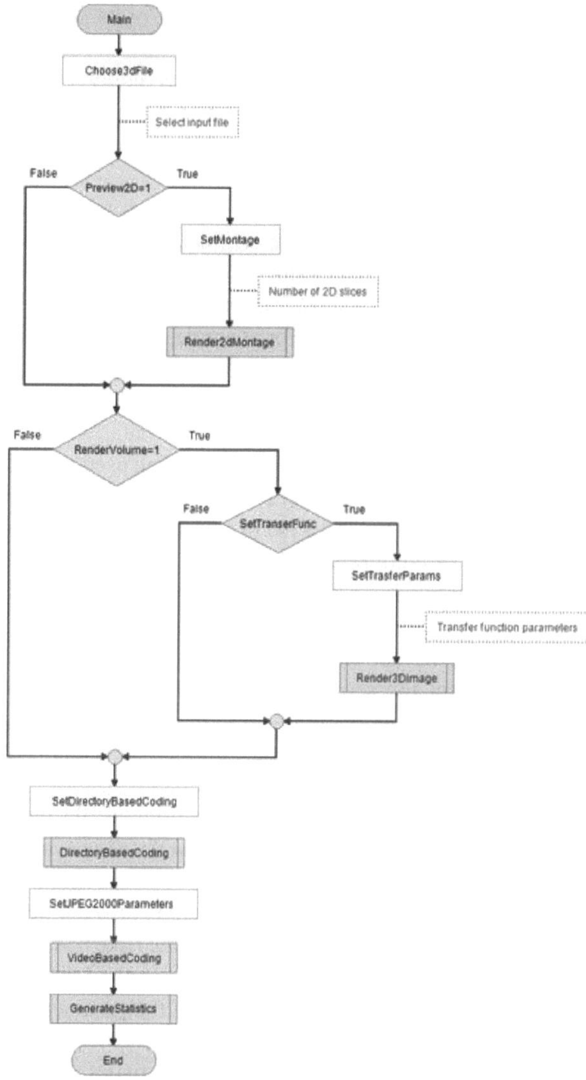

Fig. 3: Flowchar of testing

The 3D medical data storage and encoding test system has the following functionalities: viewer for 2D Medical data (1 slice), montage-viewer for set of 2D medical data, free point of view volume renderer for 3D medical data, transfer function changeability for volume renderer, efficient 3D medical data storage with JPEG2000 and H264 video coding, 3D RAW data encoder and decoder.

A. Test Story-line

The 3D medical data sets are stored in the database of our test server. One 3D data set consists of slices through an object, where each 2D slice is normally presented as a grey scale image. We can view the 2D images one-by-one, or get a montage of the 2D slices (as a preview), in 9, 16, or 64 pictures in array.

In order to view the original 3D data, we apply a texture-based volume rendering technique, where we perform the sampling and compositing steps by rendering a set of slices inside the volume.

Using our volume rendering engine, we can render a free point of view 3D image from the original data set. We use an optical model to map data values to optical properties (like color and opacity). Optical parameters calculated by applying transfer functions to the data. For example, with changing the transfer function, we can render the tooth with more intensity than the surrounding bones.

For the efficient storage of 3D medical data, we applied and compared several compress methods. The used compression methods are: lzma, gzip, bz2, lzma with e parameter, and lossless jpeg2000. Our test system generates statistics from the efficiency of compression.According our test results, the jpeg2000 techniques are quite efficient for encoding medical data sets.

Because of the correlation between neighbouring slices, we can interpret the sequence of 2D slices as frames of a video stream (Fig. 20). In our test system, we generate a video from each 3D data sets, using lossless video encoding (H264 with ultrafast and veryslow presets, and ffv1).

In the test, at first, user selects the original 3D data to be processed. An optional montage of 2D slices is available, where the user sets the number of slices to be viewed. A free point-of-view volume rendered 3D image is also applicable, with some optional settings for the rendering (like parameters of the alpha blending). After choosing the applied directory-base methods (lzma, gz2 etc), and setting the parameters for JPEG-2000 and H264-based encoding, the medical data file is encoded in several different ways, and statistics are generated about the different compression methods.

B. Test Results

According to our test results, the H264 with ultrafast preset is much faster and near that efficient like the best directory-based methods. The H264 with very slow preset is more efficient compared to the directory-based methods and the j2k. Our environment also comprises a web-based GUI, so the rendering and compression steps can be controlled from the far client as well.

We investigated the JPEG-2000 file size at lossless compression compared to other lossless format (Figure 4).

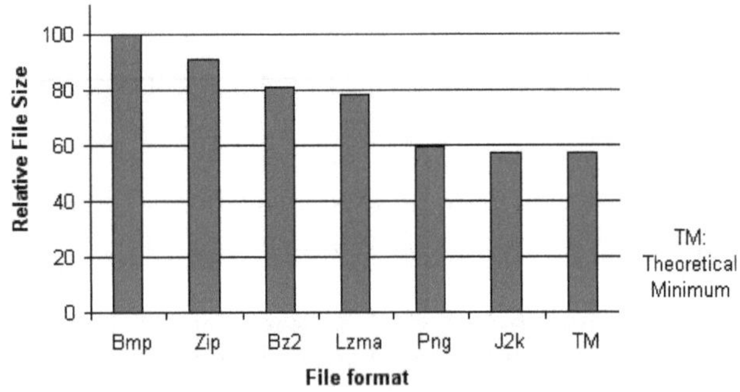

Fig. 4: File sizes at lossless compression

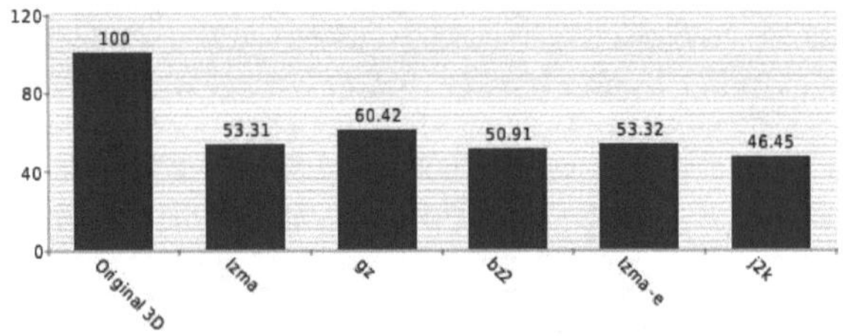

Fig. 5: Applied lossless file compressions - file sizes in percentage

According our test results, the lossless JPEG-2000 compression is more efficient then the other common compression methods (zip, lzma, bzip2...). We have calculated the Shannon-entropy of the test files (defined by $H = \sum x_i p(x_i)$ and the average code word length to find out the theoretical minimum of the lossless encoded files. The theoretically minimal file size is more than 99.99% of the j2k encoded file, so the JPEG-2000 lossless encoding could be considered quasi-optimal and practically applicable (against the Huffman-coding).

In addition to the efficient lossless compression, the JPEG-2000 techniques provide near-lossless and highly scalable lossy compression

We investigated the lossy JPEG-2000 compression file sizes at different Peak Signal to Noise Ratio (Figure 6).

At 80dB PSNR (and above) the file size is about equal to the lossless compressed file (theoretically inf PSNR). So if the medical application requires at least 80dB PSNR, the lossless compression is more relevant.

Under 40dB PSNR the degradation of quality makes the compressed file useless. Between 40 and 80 dB, the file size sharply increasing (almost linearly).

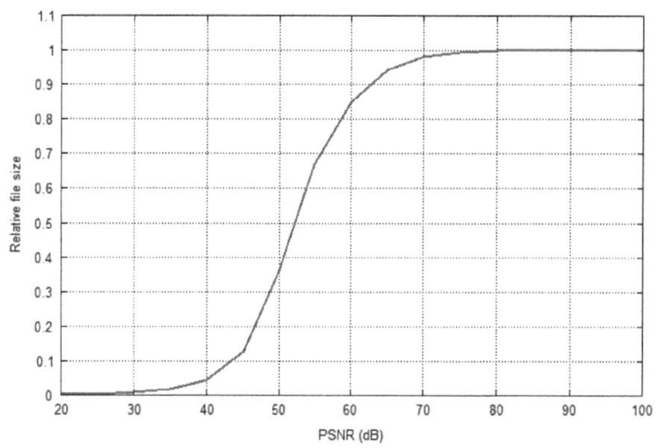

Fig. 6: Relative file size - PSNR function

We have investigated the required compression time at different PSNRs. According our measurements (fig 7), the compression time is nearly independent of the PSNR (constant).

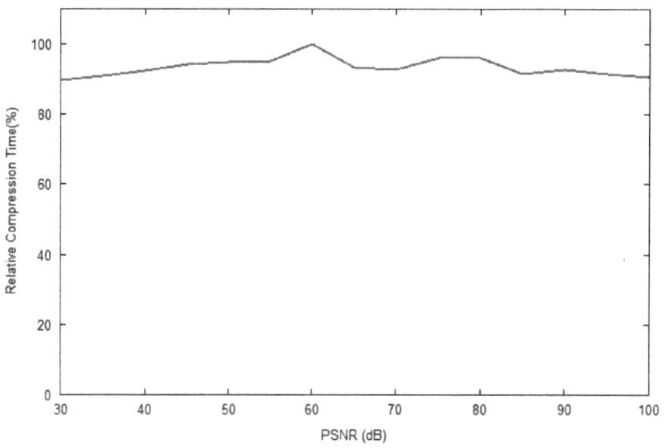

Fig. 7: Compression time - PSNR function

There are local extreme points and increasing and decreasing intervals on the function, but the test was performed not with a dedicated machine, so fluctuations may have been caused by other background processes. It could be said that with lossy compression the compression time is irreducible.

Investigating the decompression time, we obtained a near-linear, slightly increasing tendency. Reducing the image quality, the decreasing the decompression time is significantly lower than decreasing of file size.

IV. Conclusion

We implemented a test system to investigate state-of-the-art coding technologies in DICOM stored medical data compression. The lossless coding is more effective than the other,

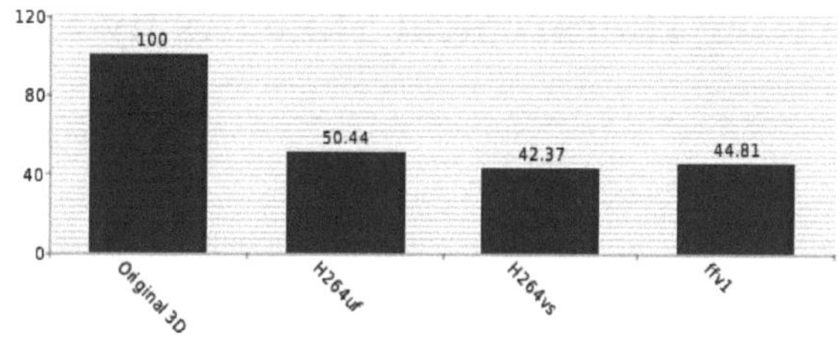

Fig. 8: Applying video coding for 3D data sets file sizes in percentage

common-used methods (like variable length coding). If an application needs at least 80 dB PSNR, the lossy coding is not appropriate. Between 40 and 80 dB, the file size sharply increasing (almost linearly). The JPEG-2000 technology is quite efficient for 3d medical data compressing.

Conflict of Interest

The authors declare that they have no conflict of interest.

Acknowledgements

The research leading to these results has received funding from the European Union's Seventh Framework Programme ([FP7/2007-2013]) under grant agreement n 288502 (Project acronym: CONCERTO). The author is grateful to the many individuals whose work made this research possible.

References

1. *DICOM. Digital Imaging and Communications in Medicine (DICOM): Part 5 Data Structures and Extensions*, 2008.
2. Tim Bruylants, Joeri Barbarien Adrian Munteanu, Jan Cornelis and Peter Schelkens, *Standardized Technologies for Volumetric Image Coding*, EEE COMSOC MMTC E-Letter (2011)
3. Taubman, D. S., and Marcellin, M. W., *JPEG2000: image compression fundamentals, standards, and practice*, Kluwer Academic Publishers, ISBN 978-0-792-37519-7 (2001).
4. ISO/IEC 15444-1 and ITU-T Rec. T.800, *Information technology JPEG 2000 image coding system: Core coding system* (2002).
5. ISO/IEC 15444-10 and ITU-T Rec. T.809, *Information technology JPEG 2000 image coding system Part 10: Extensions for three-dimensional data* (2008).
6. William A. Pearlman, *Scalable Wavelet Compression of Higher Dimension Medical Images* IEEE COMSOC MMTC E-Letter
7. David A. Clunie, *What is Different About Medical Image Compression?*, IEEE COMSOC MMTC E-Letter Vol.6, No.7, July 2011

Author: László Tóth
Institute: Budapest University of Technology and Economics
Street: Műegyetem rkp. 3.
City: Budapest
Country: Hungary
Email: tothl@hit.bme.hu

Deriving Hierarchical Statistics by Processing High Throughput Medical Images

K. Kapitány and Á. Barsi

Department of Photogrammetry and Geoinformatics, BME, Budapest, Hungary

Abstract— **This paper presents an automatic processing of high amount images of X-ray synchrotron tomographic microscopy. The developed method enables the analysis of vascular and even of microvascular network of different organs. In this study a cylindrical shaped, NiDAB labelled brain sample of a diameter of half a millimeter was imaged and analyzed with an effective pixel size of 0.38 µm. Above a thousand of tomographic slices build up the reconstructed volume meaning that an automatized analysis tool is indispensable. The developed algorithm extracts vessel cross-sections from the images and their statistics are stored in a structured format. Then the vessel reconstruction is executed, so all vessel level statistics can be derived. Having all vessels reconstructed, the tissue level features are getting available. The presented hierarchical structure of the data ensures easier connection to the data set, and supports the further medical or biological analyses of the tissue. The structure was designed to manage many tissues (evaluating multiple samples) in the similar manner.**

Keywords— **vessel analysis, high throughput data, hierarchical model, cerebral cortex, image processing**

I. INTRODUCTION

The imaging techniques of nowadays are getting more important thanks to the increasing quality, resolution and speed of image acquisition. This instrumentation is extremely important in the research of the brain, because the complexity, the functioning and diseases of this organ has been better understood. Our research aims to focus on the algorithmic development to process such imagery, special care on high throughput images. The x-ray synchrotron tomography (XRST) seems very promising, where the bright photon beam delivered by a synchrotron fulfils the researchers' requirements having also the possibility to tune the geometric resolution. [1,2] This unique equipment is very useful for the studies of the vascular system at the micrometer scale.

From the large XRST data sets it is reliable to characterize morphometric and topological characteristics of vessels networks. [3,4,5] Moreover such data provide vessel network reconstruction being a realistic basis for a numerical simulation of hemodynamics. XRST is applicable only post mortem, but it can be very important in human studies, too. XRST does not require complicated histological processing for vessel reconstruction.

II. MATERIALS AND METHODS

A. Materials

XRST images were obtained from a sample of cerebral cortex of adult marmoset (Callithrix jacchus). Animals were treated in accordance with the Guide for the Care and Use of Laboratory Animals (National Research Council 1996), European Directive 86/609 and the guidelines of the local institutional animal care and use committee.

Transcardial perfusion of an aldehyde solution was applied to preserve brain structure and the sample was treated with Avidin Biotin Complex (ABC) protocol (Elite kit, Vector Laboratoires, Burlingame, CA 94010, USA) and nickel-intensified diaminobenzidine (NiDAB; Sigma-Aldrich, Saint-Quentin Fallavier, France) as the chromogen. [6] After the NiDAB reaction, the sample was osmicated (1% OsO_4, (Electron Microscopy Sciences, Hatfield, PA 19440, USA) and 5% sucrose in PB for 60 minutes). It was also dehydrated and infiltrated with resin as described above. In order to contrast x-ray-imaged vessels, barium sulfate solution was perfused in the general blood circulation in advance of the transcardial perfusion, according to the protocol described in Plouraboué et al. (2004) and Risser et al. (2009). [7,4]

B. Methods

The sample was imaged at the TOMCAT beamline [2] of the Swiss Light Source at the Paul Scherrer Institut in Switzerland. Monochromatic synchrotron x-rays were used for the probing radiation with an energy of 10 keV (wavelength of 0.12 nm). The x-ray beam traversing the sample produces shadow images that were recorded by a CCD camera coupled with a microscopic objective of 20× magnification. The effective pixel size was 0.38 µm. The specimen was rotated during acquisition with the axis perpendicular to the x-ray beam direction. With 1501 radiographic projections the angular range of 180 degrees was covered in an equidistant manner to obtain tomographic images. The sample consists of 2048^3 pixels covering a cylinder with a height and diameter of 780 µm both. According to the stąnce and position the unnecessary images were removed. Fig. 1 shows a small detail of a tomographic slice.

Á. Jobbágy (ed.), *First European Biomedical Engineering Conference for Young Investigators*,
IFMBE Proceedings 50, DOI: 10.1007/978-981-287-573-0_8

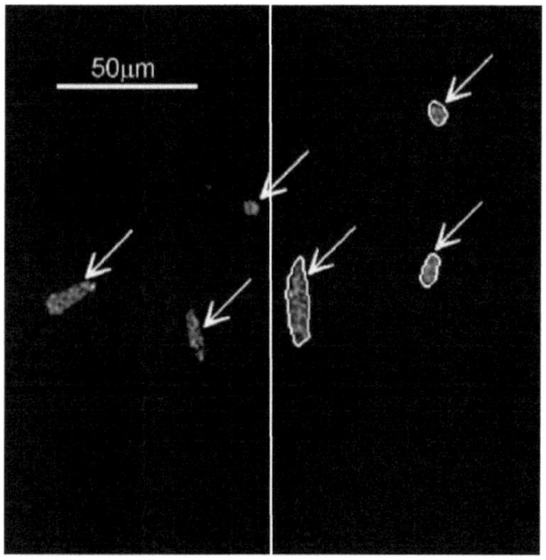

Fig. 1 Tomographic slice; Arrows point to vessel cross-sections, where the outer boundaries are marked in white.

Because of the high amount data manual image processing is not an option. The presented automatic algorithm with predefined parameters could replace this labor-intensive, yet inefficient work. The parameters are depending on the sample's shape and size, the staining method and also the condition of the sample (image failures, noises etc.).

The image processing starts with the segmentation of the vessel cross-sections. The non-homogeneity of the staining is considered by the application of the local rescaled-range calculation (LRRC) technique known from texture analysis. [8] The segmentation is finished by noise filtering.

A digital "punch" technique was applied to remove the unwanted part from the detected segments [9].

The developed method supports vessel reconstruction. Statistics were collected about each vessel cross-section. If vascular network is considered as a network of cylindrical tubes, the centroid's coordinates and the matching semi-minor axis lengths of each detected cross-section are the bases to build a generalized model [10]. This is true only if the topology of the network is available, because the connections between the discrete cross-sections are required to create vessel models. In the topology determination each centroid is projected to the adjacent tomographic slices and a search radius is drawn with the length of the matching semi-minor axis around the projections on the particular slices, including the one around the centroid itself. Then detected centroids inside the projected circles are counted, and being one or more centroids inside, detected elements are connected. Each element is labeled uniquely, but with the connection between different centroids, all get the same identification number, and therefore continuous vessel branches are established. At each bifurcation the vessels are partitioned, and the labels of the sub-branches differ. Vessel ends' coordinates are handled as an additional parameter. The acquired statistics are stored in a hierarchical structure to differentiate levels for the analyzed objects (Fig. 2).

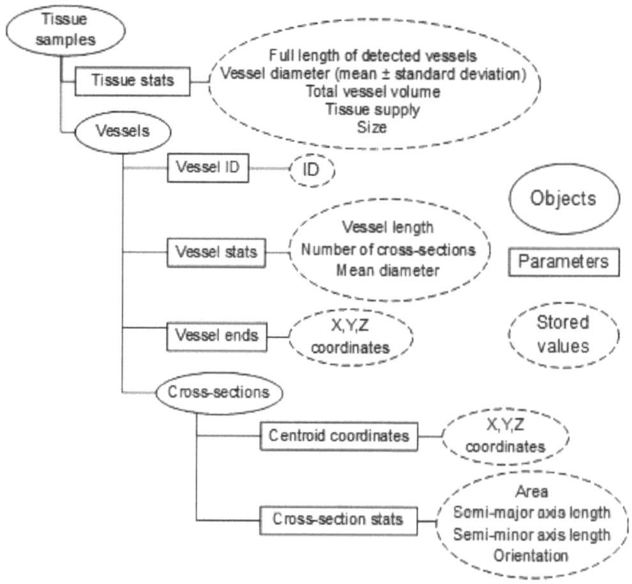

Fig. 2 Hierarchical storage of the obtained data.

This method provides opportunity to analyze the samples in general, or the connected vessels' statistics, or the vessel cross-sections separately. [10] Fig. 3 shows the whole process in flowchart, starting from the living subject and finishing by the derived and analyzed data.

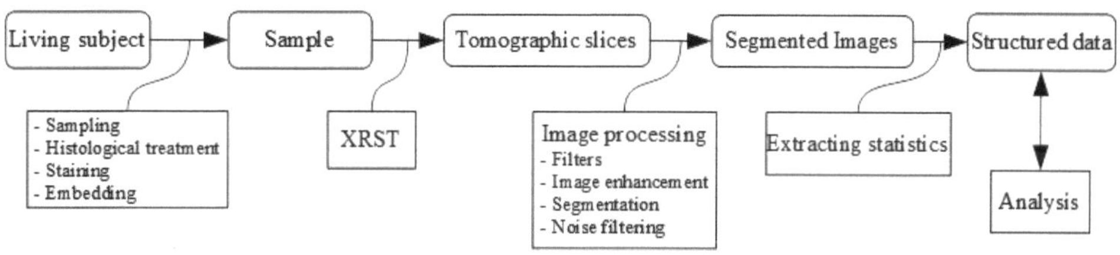

Fig. 3 Flowchart of the presented method.

III. RESULTS

The developed method has been performed on a sample processed with XRST compatible histological techniques. NiDAB staining resulted in enough parenchymal background staining, which allowed the labeling of the vessels.

The high throughput image processing including vessels reconstruction is an automated procedure taking 2378 seconds in Matlab on a regular PC. This image analysis can be interpreted as a computation speed of 2.1 sec/image.

This process time contains already the analysis of the segmented images. Statistical data is derived from each cross-section, and the parameters (area, axis lengths etc.) presented in Fig. 2 are acquired. As an example for cross-section level statistics Fig. 4 shows a distribution diagram of minor- and major-axis length of all detected segments.

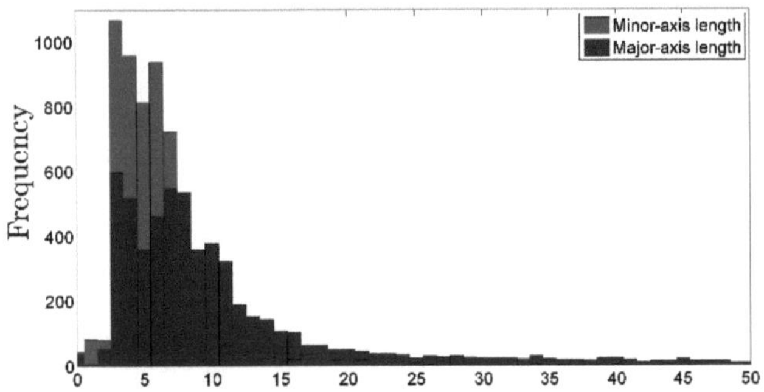

Fig. 4 Minor and major-axis length of the cross-sections [μm].

After cross-sections are analyzed and their statistics are stored in a structured format. Then the vessel reconstruction is executed, so all vessel level statistics can be derived, similarly in structured form. On this level the measures are describing the vessel segments each by each. Having all vessels reconstructed, the tissue level features are getting available. Table 1 presents statistics describing the whole sample (the tissue level) and the detected vessel structure. The calculation of statistics has been based on software and did not require any user interaction. Table 1 presents also some derived statistical features about the vascular morphometry. The total length and volume of the reconstructed vessels can be used to evaluate the tissue blood supply by calculating their ratio. Vessel volume is calculated from the number of voxels in each vessel cross-section.

The developed structure of the data ensures easier connection to the data set, and supports the further medical or biological analyses of the tissue [11]. The structure was designed to manage many tissues (evaluating multiple samples) in the similar manner.

Table 1 Tissue level statistics

Sample size (cylindrical shape, diameter × thickness) [μm]	500 × 60
Number of images	1135
Number of detected vessel cross-sections	6058
Number of detected vessel segments	934
Length of the longest vessel [μm]	69.16
Mean length of vessel segments [μm]	2.46 ± 5.82
Full length of detected vessels [μm]	2302.04
Vessel diameter (mean ± standard deviation) [μm]	3.99 ± 3.14
Median of the vessels' diameter [μm]	3.37
Volume of the examined sample [μm^3]	11 780 972
Total vessel volume [μm^3]	235 060.89
Relative volume of vessels [%]	2
Tissue supply (vessel length/ tissue volume) [$\mu m/\mu m^3$]	1.954×10^{-4}

IV. DISCUSSION AND CONCLUSION

This study describes a methodology and results of a computer based reconstruction and analysis procedure. The developed algorithm extracts information about animal brain tissue vasculature at high resolution. The applied XRST technique doesn't require complicated histological processing. The paper has been proved the evidence for the interest to use microtomography in brain tissue research, as it provides adequate information by automated processing in a reasonable time. Previous studies based on XRST of vessel used barium staining, however the complete perfusion and staining – mainly of the very fine vessel branches – has some uncertainty. The proposed image analysis technique seems to overcome of this drawback. In the study of the finest vessel network one has to test the adaptivity even in clinical conditions.

The distribution of the vessels is not homogeneous as Risser et al. [3] has shown at a small scale, whose size is close to the thickness of the sample (50-60 μm). The situation may be different from one sample to another, independently of the staining method.

Parameter changes such as vessel diameter, tortuosity and density are related to the disease in large vessels, as several papers have proven [12,13,14,15,16], few results are reported at the microscopic scale [12,17]. The development of a multiscale approach is therefore a crucial task, where innovative quantitative analysis tools are able to characterize the capillary networks in the brain and even the tracking of a disease progression is getting available.

Conflict of Interest

The authors declare that they have no conflict of interest.

References

1. Mokso R, Marone F, Irvine S, Nyvlt M, Schwyn D, Mader K, Taylor GK, Krapp HG, Skeren M, Stampanoni M (2013) Advantages of phase retrieval for fast x-ray tomographic microscopy. J. Physics D: Appl Phys. 46(49): 494004 doi:10.1088/0022-3727/46/49/494004
2. Stampanoni M, Marone F, Modregger P, Pinzer B, Thüring T, Vila-Comamala J, David C, Mokso R (2010) Tomographic hard x-ray phasecontrast micro- and nano-imaging at Tomcat. AIP Conference Proceedings, 1266: 13–17. doi: 10.1063/1.3478189
3. Risser L, Plouraboué F, Steyer A, Cloetens P, Le Duc G, Fonta C (2007) From homogeneous to fractal normal and tumorous microvascular networks in the brain. Journal of Cerebral Blood Flow and Metabolism Feb;27(2):293-303.
4. Risser L, Plouraboué F, Cloetens P, Fonta C (2009) A 3D-investigation shows that angiogenesis in primate cerebral cortex mainly occurs at capillary level. International Journal of Developmental Neuroscience Apr;27(2):185-96. doi: 10.1016/j.ijdevneu.2008.10.006.
5. Heinzer S, Krucker T, Stampanoni M, Abela R, Meyer EP, Schuler A, Schneider P, Müller R (2006) Hierarchical microimaging for multiscale analysis of large vascular networks. Neuroimage. Aug 15;32(2):626-36.
6. Negyessy L, Gal V, Farkas T, Toldi J (2000) Cross-modal plasticity of the corticothalamic circuits in rats enucleated on the first postnatal day. Eur J Neurosci. May;12(5):1654-68.
7. Plouraboué F, Cloetens P, Fonta C, Steyer A, Lauwers F, Marc-Vergnes JP (2004) High resolution X-ray imaging of vascular networks. J Microsc 215:139–148
8. Russ, John C, (1998) Image Processing Handbook, Third Edition, ISBN: 0-8493-2532-3
9. Kapitány, K (2012) Geometric reduction of high amount histological image data - A digital-punch approach. Budapest: Conference of Junior Researchers in Civil Engineering, pp. 77-82.
10. Kapitány, K (2013) Automatic generation and storage of vascular network topology. Budapest: Second Conference of Junior Researchers in Civil Engineering, pp. 1-5.
11. Kapitány K, Négyessy L, Fonta C, Mokso R, Barsi Á, Szepessy Zs (2015) Automatic reconstruction of brain's micro-vascular network based on x-ray synchrotron tomography. Biomechanica Hungarica. In press.
12. Meyer EP, Ulmann-Schuler A, Staufenbiel M, Krucker T. (2008) Altered morphology and 3D architecture of brain vasculature in a mouse model for Alzheimer's disease. Proceedings of the National Academy of Sciences of the United States of America. Mar 4;105(9):3587-92. doi: 10.1073/pnas.0709788105.
13. Dorr A, Sahota B, Chinta LV, Brown ME, Lai AY, Ma K, Hawkes CA, McLaurin J, Stefanovic B (2012) Amyloid-beta-dependent compromise of microvascular structure and function in a model of Alzheimer's disease. Brain. Oct;135(Pt 10):3039-50. doi: 10.1093/brain/aws243.
14. Biron KE, Dickstein DL, Gopaul R, Jefferies WA (2011) Amyloid triggers extensive cerebral angiogenesis causing blood brain barrier permeability and hypervascularity in Alzheimer's disease. PLoS One. 2011;6(8):e23789. doi: 10.1371/journal.pone.0023789
15. Brown WR, Thore CR. (2011) Review: cerebral microvascular pathology in ageing and neurodegeneration. Neuropathol Appl Neurobiol. Feb;37(1):56-74. doi: 10.1111/j.1365-2990.2010.01139.x.
16. Desai BS, Schneider JA, Li JL, Carvey PM, Hendey B. Evidence of angiogenic vessels in Alzheimer's disease (2009) J Neural Transm. May;116(5):587-97. doi: 10.1007/s00702-009-0226-9.
17. Klohs J, Rudin M, Shimshek DR, Beckmann N (2014) Imaging of cerebrovascular pathology in animal models of Alzheimer's disease. Frontiers in aging neuroscience Mar 13;6:32. doi: 10.3389/fnagi.2014.00032.

Author: Kristóf Kapitány
Institute: Department of Photogrammetry and Geoinformatics, BME
Street: 3 Műegyetem rkp., H-1111
City: Budapest
Country: Hungary
Email: kapitany.kristof@epito.bme.hu

Towards Multipurpose Drug Repositioning: Fusion of Multiple Kernels and Partial Equivalence Relations Using GPU-accelerated Metric Learning

B. Bolgár and P. Antal

Department of Measurement and Information Systems, Budapest University of Technology and Economics, Budapest, Hungary

Abstract— **Distance Metric Learning (DML) can be a valuable tool in biomedical data analysis as it can incorporate both partial logical equivalences and multiple similarities, solving the multitask fusion problem by producing a unified view of the entities. However, many implementations are too slow to be applied on real-world data and can benefit from GPU acceleration. Here we present and evaluate a GPU-accelerated DML framework in a drug repositioning context, where DML allows repositioning in a symmetric fashion for both drugs and diseases.**

Keywords— **Metric Learning, drug repositioning, GPGPU**

I. INTRODUCTION

A distinctive feature of biomedical data and knowledge is heterogeneity, frequently expressed in a dual form of incomplete and inconsistent equivalence relations and multiple similarities between entities of a set. This is especially true in the field of *in silico* drug discovery. Multiple chemical similarities have been employed in virtual compound screening studies for more than a decade [1]. Equivalence relations also arise naturally in a number of scenarios, *e.g.* drug combinations, interactions or shared indications. However, combining these heterogeneous data in a mathematically sound framework remained an open challenge.

A promising candidate to incorporate such dual priors is Distance Metric Learning [2], which is rooted in dimensionality reduction, and was recently extended to data fusion [3] and information geometry [4]. It can also be thought of as "inverse clustering", where a combined metric is learned from a set of base metrics with respect to prior pairwise equivalence and inequivalence relations. However, the pharmacological application of current DML implementations is hindered by the time complexity of the computations, which makes the utilization of graphics processors (GPUs) an attractive option.

In this work, first we derive a DML framework for dual priors, then discuss its parallelization and finally evaluate the GPU implementation in drug repositioning, where one aims to discover new indications for already approved drugs.

This paper is an extended version of the talk presented at the International Workshop on Technical Computing for Machine Learning and Mathematical Engineering, Leuven, 2014.

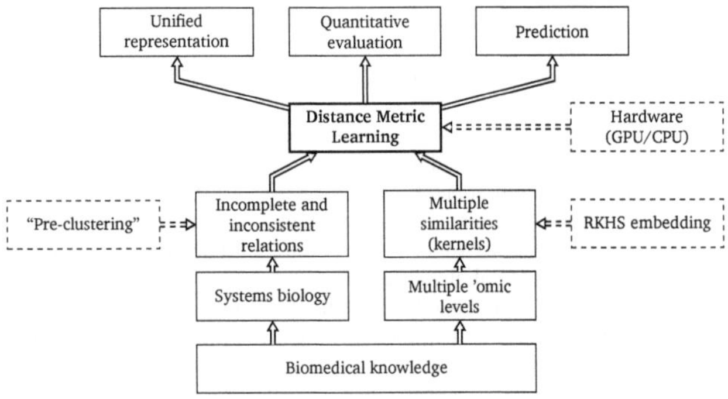

Fig. 1: An illustration of the workflow followed in this paper. DML integrates incomplete/inconsistent relations and multiple similarities stemming from the biomedical background knowledge, providing a unified view of multiple, heterogeneous information sources.

II. DISTANCE METRIC LEARNING

We aim to combine multiple metrics on flat spaces $\{\mathbb{R}^{D_k}\}_k$ given by matrices $\boldsymbol{W}_k$ corresponding to k data sources (for a related approach, see [3]). We specify training instances as $\{(\boldsymbol{x}_{ik}, \boldsymbol{z}_{ik}, y_i, C_i)\}_{i=1}^{P}$ where $\boldsymbol{x}_{ik}, \boldsymbol{z}_{ik} \in \mathbb{R}^{D_k}$ are samples in the kth data source, $y_i \in \{-1,+1\}$ denotes their relationship, and $C_i \in \mathbb{R}$ reflects our confidence in that relationship. Let d_i denote the squared distance of the two entities in the ith training instance. Since the spaces can be canonically identified with their respective tangent spaces, we can write

$$d_i = \sum_k \left\langle \boldsymbol{W}_k, (\boldsymbol{x}_{ik} - \boldsymbol{z}_{ik}) \otimes (\boldsymbol{x}_{ik} - \boldsymbol{z}_{ik}) \right\rangle_F$$

where k indexes the data sources and $\langle\cdot,\cdot\rangle_F$ is the Frobenius product. Adapting the work of Vishwanathan *et al.* [5], an analogous formulation of the metric learning problem is

$$\begin{aligned} \min_{\boldsymbol{W},\boldsymbol{m},\xi} \quad & \frac{1}{2}\sum_k \frac{\|\boldsymbol{W}_k - \boldsymbol{W}_k^0\|_F^2}{m_k} + \sum_i C_i\xi_i + \frac{\lambda}{2}\|\boldsymbol{m}\|_p^2 \\ s.t. \quad & y_i(r - d_i) \geq \rho - \xi_i, \quad \xi_i \geq 0, \quad m_k > 0, \end{aligned}$$

where $\boldsymbol{W}_k^0$ is the kth base metric, m_k is the weight of the kth data source, ξ_i's are the slack variables, C_i controls the individual contribution of training instances to the solution and overall model complexity, and the last term stands for the

Á. Jobbágy (ed.), *First European Biomedical Engineering Conference for Young Investigators*,
IFMBE Proceedings 50, DOI: 10.1007/978-981-287-573-0_9

squared L_p-norm regularization of the weights. The first constraint can be decomposed as

$$\begin{aligned}(d_i, y_i = +1) \quad &\Rightarrow \quad d_i \leq r - \rho, \\ (d_i, y_i = -1) \quad &\Rightarrow \quad d_i \geq r + \rho,\end{aligned}$$

i.e. when the entities $\boldsymbol{x}_i$, $\boldsymbol{z}_i$ are of the same class (denoted by $y_i = 1$), the distance should be small, and for dissimilar entities ($y_i = -1$) the distance should be large. The constants r and ρ control the ratio of distance between similar and dissimilar entities.

The L_2-regularized dual is derived to be

$$\begin{aligned}\max_{\boldsymbol{\alpha}} \quad & -\frac{1}{8\lambda}\sum_k \left(\boldsymbol{\alpha}^T \boldsymbol{Q}_k \boldsymbol{\alpha}\right)^2 - \sum_i \alpha_i y_i \left(r - d_i^0\right) + \boldsymbol{\rho}^T \boldsymbol{\alpha} \\ s.t. \quad & 0 \leq \alpha_i \leq C_i,\end{aligned}$$

where d_i^0 is the base distance for the ith sample and

$$\begin{aligned}\boldsymbol{q}_{ik} &= y_i \left(\boldsymbol{x}_{ik} - \boldsymbol{z}_{ik}\right) \otimes \left(\boldsymbol{x}_{ik} - \boldsymbol{z}_{ik}\right) \\ \boldsymbol{Q}_{k_{ij}} &= \left\langle \boldsymbol{q}_{ik}, \boldsymbol{q}_{jk} \right\rangle_F = y_i y_j \left\langle \left(\boldsymbol{x}_{ik} - \boldsymbol{z}_{ik}\right), \left(\boldsymbol{x}_{jk} - \boldsymbol{z}_{jk}\right) \right\rangle^2.\end{aligned}$$

We solve the convex optimization problem by using gradient projection (Algorithm 1). The squared distance of two arbitrary samples $\boldsymbol{x}$ and $\boldsymbol{z}$ can then be computed from the dual variables as

$$\sum_k \left[d_k^0(\boldsymbol{x}, \boldsymbol{z}) - m_k \sum_i \alpha_i \left\langle \boldsymbol{q}_{ik}, (\boldsymbol{x}_k - \boldsymbol{z}_k) \otimes (\boldsymbol{x}_k - \boldsymbol{z}_k) \right\rangle_F \right].$$

Utilizing the kernel PCA (KPCA) trick [6], the algorithm can be extended to the non-linear setting by parameterizing $\boldsymbol{W}_k = (\boldsymbol{F}_k \boldsymbol{\Phi}_k)^T \boldsymbol{F}_k \boldsymbol{\Phi}_k$, so that

$$\begin{aligned}d_i &= \sum_k \left\| \boldsymbol{F}_k \boldsymbol{\Phi}_k (\phi_k(\boldsymbol{x}_{ik}) - \phi_k(\boldsymbol{z}_{ik})) \right\|_F^2 \\ &= \sum_k \left\langle \boldsymbol{F}_k^T \boldsymbol{F}_k, (\tilde{\boldsymbol{x}}_{ik} - \tilde{\boldsymbol{z}}_{ik}) \otimes (\tilde{\boldsymbol{x}}_{ik} - \tilde{\boldsymbol{z}}_{ik}) \right\rangle_F,\end{aligned}$$

where $\boldsymbol{\Phi}$ is the matrix $[\phi_k(\boldsymbol{x}_{1k})\ \phi_k(\boldsymbol{x}_{2k})\ \cdots\ \phi_k(\boldsymbol{x}_{nk})]^T$ and thus the transformed samples $\tilde{\boldsymbol{x}}$ correspond to the rows of a suitable Gram matrix.

III. GPU Implementation

The main steps are shown in Algorithm 1. Computing the transformed representations in Step 2 is essentially the same as computing the Gram matrix, which is usually a compute-bound operation and can be performed very efficiently by using modified General Matrix Multiplication (GEMM) routines. Modified sparse routines were also implemented for

Algorithm 1 Parallel gradient projection for metric learning.

// Initialization:
1: **for** all k **do**
2: Compute $\widetilde{\boldsymbol{X}}_k = [\tilde{\boldsymbol{x}}_{ik}]$ **in parallel.**
3: Compute $\widetilde{\boldsymbol{X}}_k \widetilde{\boldsymbol{X}}_k^T$ **in parallel.**
4: **for** all i **do in parallel**
5: Compute $d_i^0 = \sum_k \left\langle \boldsymbol{I}_k, (\tilde{\boldsymbol{x}}_{ik} - \tilde{\boldsymbol{z}}_{ik}) \otimes (\tilde{\boldsymbol{x}}_{ik} - \tilde{\boldsymbol{z}}_{ik}) \right\rangle_F = \sum_k \|\tilde{\boldsymbol{x}}_{ik} - \tilde{\boldsymbol{z}}_{ik}\|_2^2.$
6: Initialize $\boldsymbol{\alpha} \leftarrow 0, \quad (\boldsymbol{\alpha}^T \boldsymbol{Q}_k \boldsymbol{\alpha}) \leftarrow 0, \quad (\boldsymbol{Q}_k \boldsymbol{\alpha})_i \leftarrow 0.$
// Main loop:
7: **while** $\boldsymbol{\alpha}$ not optimal **do**
8: **for** all i **do**
9: **for** all k **do**
10: **for** all j **do in parallel**
11: Compute $\boldsymbol{Q}_{k_{ij}} = y_i y_j \langle \tilde{\boldsymbol{x}}_{ik} - \tilde{\boldsymbol{z}}_{ik}, \tilde{\boldsymbol{x}}_{jk} - \tilde{\boldsymbol{z}}_{jk} \rangle^2.$
// Gradient projection:
12: Compute $A = \frac{1}{2\lambda} \sum_k \boldsymbol{Q}_{k_{ii}}^2.$
13: Compute $B = \frac{3}{2\lambda} \sum_k \boldsymbol{Q}_{k_{ii}} (\boldsymbol{Q}_k \boldsymbol{\alpha})_i.$
14: Compute $C = \frac{1}{2\lambda} \left(\sum_k \boldsymbol{Q}_{k_{ii}} \boldsymbol{\alpha}^T \boldsymbol{Q}_k \boldsymbol{\alpha} + 2((\boldsymbol{Q}_k \boldsymbol{\alpha})_i)^2 \right).$
15: Compute $D = \sum_k m_k (\boldsymbol{Q}_k \boldsymbol{\alpha})_i + y_i(r - d_i^0) - \rho.$
16: $\delta \leftarrow$ largest root of $A\delta^3 + B\delta^2 + C\delta + D = 0$ projected into the feasible region.
17: $\alpha_i \leftarrow \alpha_i + \delta.$
// Update caches:
18: **for** all k **do**
19: $(\boldsymbol{\alpha}^T \boldsymbol{Q}_k \boldsymbol{\alpha}) \leftarrow (\boldsymbol{\alpha}^T \boldsymbol{Q}_k \boldsymbol{\alpha}) + \boldsymbol{Q}_{k_{ii}} \delta^2 + 2(\boldsymbol{Q}_k \boldsymbol{\alpha})_i \delta.$
20: $m_k \leftarrow \frac{1}{2\lambda} \boldsymbol{\alpha}^T \boldsymbol{Q}_k \boldsymbol{\alpha}.$
21: **for** all k, j **do in parallel**
22: $(\boldsymbol{Q}_k \boldsymbol{\alpha})_j \leftarrow (\boldsymbol{Q}_k \boldsymbol{\alpha})_j + \boldsymbol{Q}_{k_{ij}} \delta.$

sparse matrices using the Expansion–Sorting–Compression method. However, the full matrix might not fit into the memory; in this case, the KPCA trick is taken a step further by performing the dimensionality reduction.

It is clear from the derivation that the values of $\boldsymbol{Q}_k$ depend solely on inner products, moreover, if we set $\boldsymbol{W}_k^0 \leftarrow \boldsymbol{I}$, base distances in Step 5 can also be computed from the same inner products. Therefore, in Step 3, a GEMM operation is performed to compute $\widetilde{\boldsymbol{X}}_k \widetilde{\boldsymbol{X}}_k^T$ and the original matrix is discarded. Again, if the full matrix does not fit into the memory, only the diagonal is computed and the rest is done on-the-fly.

In each iteration, most of the time is taken up by Steps 9-11 and 21-22, which are also ideal candidates for parallelization, since the values here can be computed independently us-

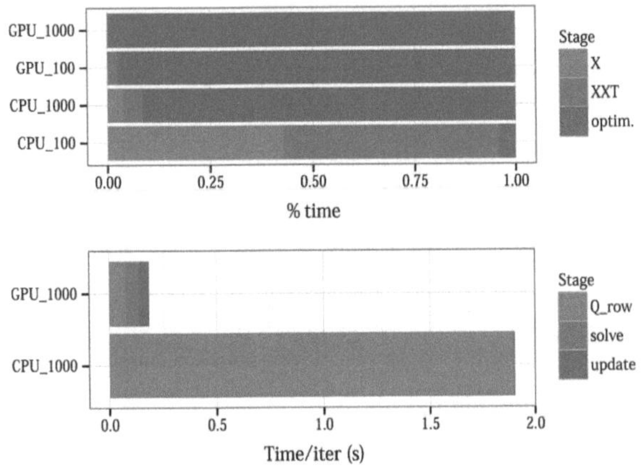

Fig. 2: The upper diagram shows the percentage of time taken up by the initialization and the optimization using 4 information sources. For a training set of 100 constraints, the actual optimization is completed much faster than the initialization on the CPU. For larger training sets, the time complexity is dominated by the optimization steps in both cases. The overall performance is depicted on Fig. 3. The lower diagram illustrates the amount of time taken up by an iteration for a training set of 1000 constraints. It is clear that the GPU is much slower in sequential operations than the CPU, however, the time complexity is dominated by the parallelized steps.

Table 1: AUC values for the multi-class (DML) and one-class (SVM) models.

Description	AUC (DML)	AUC (SVM)
selective beta blockers	**0.983**	0.831
SSRIs	0.944	**0.999**
other antiepileptics	0.875	**0.914**
protease inhibitors	**0.984**	0.920
5HT-1 agonists	0.916	**1**
Tyr kinase inhibitors	**0.968**	0.785
pyrimidine analogues	0.949	**0.995**
anthracyclines	0.957	**0.998**
NRTIs	0.911	**0.996**
other antidepressants	**0.922**	0.718
fluoroquinolones	0.**967**	0.923
ARBs	0.945	**0.999**
3rd gen cephalosporins	0.932	**0.997**
ACE inhibitors	0.899	**0.93**
Average	**0.939**	0.929

ing custom compute kernels. Steps 12-17 involve a loop over only k and therefore are performed sequentially (note that typically $k \ll j$). Similarly, Steps 18-20 require only $5k$ memory accesses, which are again done sequentially on the GPU in order to avoid unnecessary data transfer. Finally, Steps 21-22 are performed in parallel with respect to j using custom compute kernels. The time taken up by the subtasks is depicted on Fig. 2.

IV. Benchmark

Benchmark runs were carried out on a Ubuntu 14.04 desktop machine with 8GB RAM, AMD Radeon HD7970 GPU and Intel Core i5-2500K CPU, using the Eigen library for the baseline implementation [7]. Each test was run 3 times with average times reported. The algorithm yielded identical results on the CPU and GPU while the latter maintained a solid $10\times$ performance improvement for smaller training sets and around $100\times$ for larger ones. Scaling with respect to the number of information sources was also investigated. Results are summarized on Fig. 3.

V. Experiments

DML offers a natural way to find new drugs for a given indication, or *vice versa*, to find novel applications for a given drug by aggregating distances to drug class members. The predictive performance was assessed in a multiclass context. The following information sources were used:

- Chemical structure: MACCS, MolconnZ and 3D pharmacophore-based molecular descriptors, using the Tanimoto similarity measure.
- Side-effect profiles taken from the SIDER database [8] and mined from package inserts, using the cosine similarity measure.
- Target profiles obtained from the DrugBank database [9], using the cosine similarity measure.

All information were readily available from a previous work [10]. Drug class memberships were obtained from the ATC classification of drugs. The evaluation was performed in a $100\times$ 70-30 cross-validation setting as follows:

- The training set consisted of a randomly selected 70% of 100 drugs for which all information were available.
- Constraints were generated for each drug:
  - · Equivalence: 3 farthest in-class drugs (in the original Euclidean sense),
  - · Inequivalence: 5 closest out-of-class drugs.
- The remaining 30% of samples were used to compute the area under the receiver operating characteristic curve (AUC) for each class, based on average distance to in-class training samples.

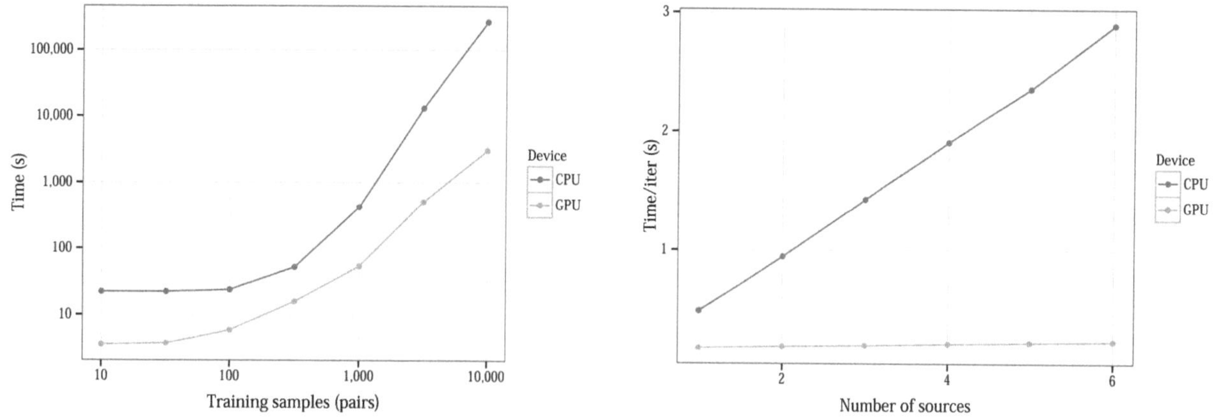

Fig. 3: The figure on the left shows the scaling properties of the CPU and GPU implementations with respect to the size of the training set. For training set sizes around 10^4, the performance improvement is two orders of magnitude. The right side shows linear scaling with respect to the number of information sources, using a training set of 1000 constraints. All computations were performed using double precision.

AUC values were compared to the values obtained in an earlier work which utilized one-class Multiple Kernel Support Vector Machines (MK-SVMs) for drug prioritization [10]. Results are shown on Table 1. It should be noted that this comparison is biased, since the SVM-based method is strictly one-class and it is a well-known fact that in the absence of negative class information, AUC tends to overestimate predictive performance [11]. Moreover, while the one-class SVM learns a separate model for each ranking task, DML learns an overall multipurpose model: the resulting metric can be used both for drug prioritization for any disease and for disease prioritization for any drug. Even so, the DML-based multi-class model yields comparable performance to that of the earlier one-class SVM-based model.

VI. Conclusion

The proposed metric learning framework provides a principled way to integrate heterogeneous background knowledge into an adaptive, consistent, unified view of the entities, while the utilization of the GPU offers a significant performance improvement.

Conflict of Interest

The authors declare that they have no conflict of interest.

Acknowledgements

Supported by OTKA112915, János Bolyai Research Scholarship of the Hungarian Academy of Sciences (P.Antal).

References

1. Ginn CMR, Willett P, Bradshaw J. Combination of molecular similarity measures using data fusion *Perspectives in Drug Discovery and Design.* 2000;20:1-16.
2. Bellet A, Habrard A, Sebban M. A Survey on Metric Learning for Feature Vectors and Structured Data *CoRR.* 2013;abs/1306.6709.
3. Wang S, Huang Q, Jiang S, Tian Q. Efficient Lp-norm Multiple Feature Metric Learning for Image Categorization in *Proceedings of the 20th ACM International Conference on Information and Knowledge Management*(New York, NY, USA):2077–2080ACM 2011.
4. Hauberg S, Freifeld O, Black MJ. A Geometric take on Metric Learning in *Advances in Neural Information Processing Systems 25*:2024–2032Curran Associates, Inc. 2012.
5. Vishwanathan SVN, Sun Z, Ampornpunt N, Varma M. Multiple Kernel Learning and the SMO Algorithm in *NIPS*:2361-2369Curran Associates, Inc. 2010.
6. Chatpatanasiri R, Kijsirikul B. A Unified Semi-supervised Dimensionality Reduction Framework for Manifold Learning *Neurocomput..* 2010;73:1631–1640.
7. Guennebaud Gaël, Jacob Benoît, others . Eigen v3 http://eigen.tuxfamily.org 2010.
8. Kuhn M, Campillos M, Letunic I, Jensen LJ, Bork P. A side effect resource to capture phenotypic effects of drugs *Mol. Syst. Biol..* 2010;6.343.
9. Law V., Knox C., Djoumbou Y., et al. DrugBank 4.0: shedding new light on drug metabolism *Nucleic Acids Res..* 2014;42:D1091–1097.
10. Arany A, Bolgar B, Balogh B, Antal P, Matyus P. Multi-aspect Candidates for Repositioning: Data Fusion Methods Using Heterogeneous Information Sources *Curr. Med. Chem..* 2013;20:95–107.
11. Rider AK, Johnson RA, Davis DA, Hoens TR, Chawla NV. Classifier Evaluation with Missing Negative Class Labels in *IDA*;8207 of *Lecture Notes in Computer Science*:380-391Springer 2013.

Author: Bence Bolgár
Institute: Dpt. of Meas. and Inf. Sys., Budapest Univ. of Tech. and Econ.
Street: Magyar tudosok krt. 2.
City: Budapest
Country: Hungary
Email: bolgar@mit.bme.hu

Decomposition of Shared Latent Factors Using Bayesian Multi-morbidity Dependency Maps

P. Marx[1,2] and P. Antal[1]

[1] Budapest University of Technology and Economics /Department of Measurement and Information Systems, Budapest, Hungary
[2] MTA-SE Neuropsychopharmacology and Neurochemistry Research Group, Budapest, Hungary

***Abstract*—The use of multiple diseases and complex phenotypic descriptors is a new trend of genetic association analysis, motivated by the pathway diseases and network medicine paradigms. Comorbidity information is an important resource in this exploration of shared molecular background. To extend the current pairwise, correlation based methods, we investigate a systems-based approach for the use of separated large-scale multi-morbidity data to explore common latent factors of related diseases. We constructed a multi-morbidity dataset from the UK Biobank by filtering rare diseases. In the first phase of our method, we use a Markov Chain Monte Carlo method over Bayesian networks to construct a Bayesian dependency map, which is confounded with many known factors. In the second phase, the method could incorporate prior causal information between the diseases and information about the known confounding by demographic, medical, genetic, environmental factors. The difference between the known causal and confounding relations and the observed dependencies is used to bind the extent of further latent factors. This reconstruction of the shared latent factors happens hierarchically in a top-down fashion, terminating with the identification of latent factors for pair of diseases. We compare our method with other comorbidity methods and systems-based network approaches in the field of psychiatry, focusing on depression and anxiety. We demonstrate the use of molecular, symptomatic and environmental knowledge bases to interpret the reconstructed latent factors. This research has been conducted using the UK Biobank Resource.**

***Keywords*—multi-morbidity, confounding, Bayesian networks, Monte Carlo methods**

I. INTRODUCTION

Between the classical clinical disease/syndrome/symptom levels and the levels of the measured molecular entities, such as genetic/epigenetic variations or genomic/proteomic/metabolomic expression data an autonomous, intermediate level emerged, the level of pathways. A working definition of pathway is an autonomous, functionally or even anatomically related set of entities, above heterogeneous, high-dimensional "omic" levels [1]. The pathway concept is essential in high-dimensional statistical analysis to cope with multiple hypothesis testing by aggregating and fostering statistically weak results over the omic variables, their molecular background are characterized by multiple results of network medicine, and in many cases, they also help to refine or even redefine clinical diseases, e.g. "pathway diseases" in cancer and psychiatry [2], [3]. Further indirect, but very fruitful results corroborating the pathway disease concepts in psychiatry were reported in genetic association analysis, based on the usage of multiple diseases with hypothetically overlapping pathways [4], [5].

In this paper we investigate a method based on the hypothesis that comorbidity information could also be used to explore pathways, especially shared pathways between multiple diseases. Note that this clinical level information source is expectably complementary to molecular omic information sources.

Comorbidity, or more precisely multi-morbidity is a common condition, more frequent than the presence of a single disease [6][7]. Its formal modeling is very challenging as the standardized description of the phenome is still lacking in clinical practice and as the causal relations between the diseases are confounded by inherent nosologic problems [8] and limitless hidden variables, such as genetic, demographic, treatment, lifestyle or environmental conditions [9].

Despite its limitations, multi-morbidity data became a standard information source to explore disease—disease relations, although only in the pairwise framework [10], [11]. Validations were based on molecular bases as well on progression of complex disease conditions [11]. A particularly relevant application for our approach used the comorbidity pairwise relations to explore the number and type of genetic factors behind pairwise interactions of diseases [10].

However, a multivariate, systems-based approach is an open challenge, although wide-range of methodological repertoire could be adapted or scaled-up in case of available data sets, such as causal Bayesian networks [12][13]. Using a manually aggregated UK Biobank data set we report preliminary results about the performance of a two-stage Bayesian, systems-based approach for exploring multi-shared common factors between diseases.

Á. Jobbágy (ed.), *First European Biomedical Engineering Conference for Young Investigators*,
IFMBE Proceedings 50, DOI: 10.1007/978-981-287-573-0_10

II. DATA

The UK Biobank contains environmental, epidemiological and genetic information. For this analysis we used a subset of the UK Biobank data (UKB) which contains 117803 patients' basic environmental and medical history. In this study, we used age, gender and body mass index (BMI) together with self-reported patient history which was processed by experts. The answers were assigned to 525 different diseases in two major groups cancer- and non-cancer illnesses. Many diseases seems to be underrepresented compared to the expected penetrance. Patients were defined obese if the respective BMI were higher than 30. As the youngest participant was 45 years old we assumed that the reported diseases reflect lifetime medical history, although this is only raw approximation even in our focus on psychiatry. After filtering all rare diseases (less than 0.1 percent of all samples) and all samples without any disease 250 disease remained. This dataset were used together with gender in the main part of the analysis.

III. METHODS

Bayesian networks provide a standard framework for the representation of probabilistic dependencies and independencies at a multivariate, global level, i.e. a dependency map through d-separation [12][14]. Furthermore, the representation supports the use of interventional data [15] and various causal interpretations (for the Causal Markov Assumption, see e.g. [16], for special approaches to cope with hidden, confounding variables, see [17]for functional Bayesian networks, see [12]). Additionally, the dynamic Bayesian network extension allows the use of temporal data.

To create a framework, which can cope with the high number of diseases, the interventional and temporal aspects, rare diseases and supports the incorporation of wide range prior information we developed a two-phased system. In the first phase, it uses Bayesian network representation in the Bayesian statistical framework to produce a Bayesian dependency map, which is analyzed in the second phase to explore shared hidden factors confounding multiple observed variables.

A. Estimation of a Bayesian Multi-morbidity Dependency Map

In this work, we neglect the onset information of the diseases and potential multiple occurrences, thus we use only a binary representation for their occurrence. We estimated the a posteriori probabilities of edges in the Bayesian network using a Markov Chain Monte Carlo method with 100,000 burn-in steps and 1,000,000 sampling steps [18][19].

B. Approximation of the number of latent factors

Because of confounding, disease connections could be the consequence of multiple, independent latent factors. To approximate the number of latent factors for a disease group connected with edges with *a posteriori* probabilities above a threshold we estimate the probabilities of hidden structures, specifically we compute the probability for the lack of confounding assuming independence for effects of the latent factors. This is illustrated for a pair of diseases D1, D2, in which case we compute the probability of the complete lack of paths leading from one disease to the other through latent factors:

$$1 - P(Edge(D_1 D_2)|DN) = \prod_{i=1}^{k} (1 - p_f^2 q), \quad (1)$$

where the probability of the edge between the diseases is $P(Edge(D_1, D_2)|DN)$, q is the general *a priori* probability of the manifestation of a latent factor and p_f is a general *a priori* probability of an edge from a latent factor to a disease. This formula is used to compute the number of latent factors behind unexplained, confounded relations.

In this study we leave open the interpretation of latent factors and treat them as pathways representing genetic, proteomic, but even environmental aspects.

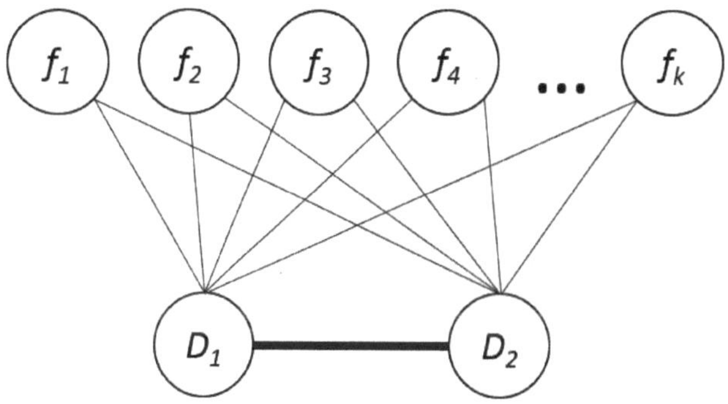

Figure 1 Independent latent factors affecting disease-disease co-morbidity

C. Latent factors for multi-morbid diseases

To extend the previously described latent factor approximation we developed a top-down algorithm, which recursively finds maximally shared latent factors confounding diseases groups.

The algorithm in Fig.2 estimates the number of latent factors based on the smallest edge of the given clique and considers these factors as the explained set of the causes creating the multi-morbid disease group.

IV. RESULTS

We applied our method to the UK Biobank self-reported patient data set with the described preprocessing steps. The resulting edges were used to approximate the number of hidden factors k. For k approximation two different methods were applied. In the first case we assumed constant effect for all factors ($p_f = 0.1$). In the second case we sampled a uniform distribution on the $[0,0.2]$ interval at every extension of the latent factors. Both resulted in an average of $\overline{p_f} = 0.1$. $q = 0.15$ *a priori* probability was used in both cases. The constant p_f resulted $k = 505$ for the depression and anxiety edge ($P(depression, anxiety)|DN) = 0.531402$). Figure 3 shows the estimated number of latent factors with prior 0.15 and uniform $\overline{p_f}$.

We collected the Bayes network edge data for mental- and mood disorders. This resulted in 3 3-cliques, all containing 'depression' and 'nervous breakdown' and one of 'manic/bipolar disorder', 'anxiety/panic attack' and 'post-natal depression'. Results showed in Table 1.

To attenuation of indirect, transitive effects in pairwise, correlational approaches, a "silencing" operation was proposed [20]. We tested the silencing method suggested for subtracting indirect effects on the odds ratio matrix with the 251 variables and compared its result with the result of our inherently systems-based method, i.e. we compared the BN edge posteriors, standard OR (odds ratio with 0.95 confidence intervals) and silenced OR matrices with Spearman rank correlation.. The mean pairwise correlation was the highest between the OR and BN edge matrices (0.139). The original OR compared with the silenced OR gave a 0.0078 rank correlation while the BN edge has an average correlation with the silenced OR of 0.0964.

Table 1 Clique result showing only the 3rd member of every clique. $p_f = 0.1$ was used in all settings. k was approximated without prior/with prior 0.15

Clique	Total k
Anxiety	646/4307
Bipolar disorder	7/43
Post-natal depression	320/2130

Begin:
1. *Find n-cliques in the Bayesian network*
2. *For every clique:*
   - *2.1. Order the disease pairs of the clique by edge weight*
   - *2.2. Compute k based on (1) for the smallest edge*
3. *Repeat for n-1-cliques*

End

Figure 2 Recursive latent factor decomposition.

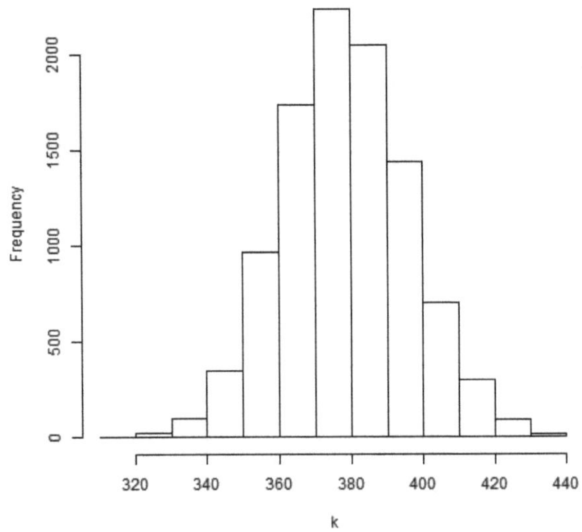

Figure 3 The estimated number of latent factors for 10000 runs.

V. DISCUSSION

Many efforts have been made to build disease—disease networks[21] for different purposes e.g. drug repositioning, finding new drug targets, co-morbidity networks, new candidate genes. These networks use similar databases or measurement techniques facing the same issues. Text-mining results are biased as many tools are context independent. GWA studies usually suffer from low sample size causing many not replicable hits. Differentially expressed genes not always imply causality. These problems often lead to transitive connections although there is a direct edge between the two diseases.

Our goal was to decipher these connections using a Bayesian, multivariate, systems-based approach and explore the number of independent shared latent factors, pathways between groups and pairs of diseases.

The systems-based approaches expectably provides more parsimonious results, but their characteristics is unexplored because of their high computational complexity. The silencing method showed decreased OR between many of the disease pairs, however the correlation with the BN method remained low. Further validation needed to understand the differences between the BN and the "silencing" results.

VI. Conclusions

The proposed model showed promising results and could be the starting point of further analysis. We are working on the following extensions: using clusters of confounded variables, instead of cliques, better approximation formulas for the hierarchical structure of latent structures and taking into account the differences between different types of latent factors (genetic, environmental etc.). With better models and the incorporation of prior knowledge about known hidden factors this Bayesian approach could lead to the discovery of hidden factors causing multi-morbid diseases, whose interpretation is another open research question.

Acknowledgment

This research was conducted in cooperation with research teams of Dr. Gabriella Juhász and Prof. Dr. György Bagdy. The authors thank their support and personal contributions.

This research has been conducted using the UK Biobank Resource. This study has been supported by National Development Agency (KTIA_NAP_13-1-2013-0001), Hungarian Brain Research Program - Grant No. KTIA_13_NAP-A-II/14, MTA-SE Neuropsychopharmacology and Neurochemistry Research Group, Hungarian Academy of Sciences, Semmelweis University, MTA-SE-NAP B Genetic Brain Imaging Migraine Research Group (8825), Hungarian Academy of Sciences, Semmelweis University, OTKA 112915, and the János Bolyai Research Scholarship of the Hungarian Academy of Sciences (P. Antal).

Conflict of Interest

The authors declare that they have no conflict of interest.

References

[1] P. F. Sullivan, M. J. Daly, and M. O'Donovan, "Genetic architectures of psychiatric disorders: the emerging picture and its implications.," *Nat. Rev. Genet.*, vol. 13, no. 8, pp. 537–51, Aug. 2012.

[2] J. W. Smoller, "Identifi cation of risk loci with shared eff ects on fi ve major psychiatric disorders: A genome-wide analysis," *Lancet*, vol. 381, no. 12, pp. 1371–1379, 2013.

[3] P. F. Sullivan, "Puzzling over schizophrenia: Schizophrenia as a pathway disease," *Nat. Med.*, vol. 18, no. 2, pp. 210–211, 2012.

[4] J. M. Shulman and P. L. De Jager, "Evidence for a common pathway linking neurodegenerative diseases.," *Nat. Genet.*, vol. 41, no. 12, pp. 1261–2, Dec. 2009.

[5] P. Network, "Psychiatric genome-wide association study analyses implicate neuronal, immune and histone pathways," *Nat. Neurosci.*, 2015.

[6] E. Capobianco and P. Lio', "Comorbidity: A multidimensional approach," *Trends Mol. Med.*, vol. 19, no. 9, pp. 515–521, 2013.

[7] K. Barnett, S. W. Mercer, M. Norbury, G. Watt, S. Wyke, and B. Guthrie, "Epidemiology of multimorbidity and implications for health care, research, and medical education: A cross-sectional study," *Lancet*, vol. 380, no. 9836, pp. 37–43, 2012.

[8] X. Zhou, J. Menche, A.-L. Barabási, and A. Sharma, "Human symptoms-disease network.," *Nat. Commun.*, vol. 5, no. May, p. 4212, Jan. 2014.

[9] U. Vaidyanathan, C. J. Patrick, and W. G. Iacono, "Patterns of comorbidity among mental disorders: a person-centered approach.," *Compr. Psychiatry*, vol. 52, no. 5, pp. 527–535, 2011.

[10] L. Yao and A. Rzhetsky, "Quantitative systems-level determinants of human genes targeted by successful drugs," *Genome Res.*, vol. 18, pp. 206–213, 2008.

[11] C. a Hidalgo, N. Blumm, A.-L. Barabási, and N. a Christakis, "A dynamic network approach for the study of human phenotypes.," *PLoS Comput. Biol.*, vol. 5, no. 4, p. e1000353, Apr. 2009.

[12] J. Pearl, "Causality: Models, Reasoning, and Inference," 2000.

[13] E. Capobianco and P. Lio, "Comorbidity networks: beyond disease correlations," *J. Complex Networks*, pp. 1–14, 2015.

[14] H. Tost and A. Meyer-Lindenberg, "Puzzling over schizophrenia: Schizophrenia, social environment and the brain," *Nat. Med.*, vol. 18, no. 2, pp. 211–213, 2012.

[15] G. F. Cooper and C. Yoo, "Causal Discovery from a Mixture of Experimental and Observational Data," in *Proc. of the 15th Conf. on Uncertainty in Artificial Intelligence ({UAI}-1999)*, 1999, pp. 116–125.

[16] C. Glymour and G. F. Cooper, *Computation, Causation, and Discovery*. AAAI Press, 1999.

[17] G. Cooper, "A simple constraint-based algorithm for efficiently mining observational databases for causal relationships," *Data Min. Knowl. Discov.*, vol. 2, pp. 203–224, 1997.

[18] D. Madigan, S. A. Andersson, M. Perlman, and C. T. Volinsky, "Bayesian model averaging and model selection for Markov equivalence classes of acyclic digraphs," *Comm.Statist. Theory Methods*, vol. 25, pp. 2493–2520, 1996.

[19] P. Antal and a Millinghoffer, "A Bayesian view of challenges in feature selection: multilevel analysis, feature aggregation, multiple targets, redundancy and interaction," *JMLR Work. ...*, no. 4, pp. 74–89, 2008.

[20] B. Barzel and A.-L. Barabási, "Network link prediction by global silencing of indirect correlations.," *Nat. Biotechnol.*, vol. 31, no. 8, pp. 720–5, 2013.

[21] A.-L. Barabási, N. Gulbahce, and J. Loscalzo, "Network medicine: a network-based approach to human disease.," *Nat. Rev. Genet.*, vol. 12, no. 1, pp. 56–68, Jan. 2011.

Author: Peter Antal
Institute: Budapest University of Technology and Economics /Department of Measurement and Information Systems, Budapest, Hungary
Street: Magyar Tudosok krt 2.
City: Budapest
Country: Hungary
Email: antal@mit.bme.hu

Bootstrap-Based Quality Scores for NGS Variant Calling

P. Sarkozy, Á. Jobbágy, and P. Antal

Budapest University of Technology and Economics, Department of Measurement and Information Systems, Budapest, Hungary

Abstract— **Variant calling, the identification of DNA sites that differ from a reference sequence using Next Generation Sequencing (NGS) methods is still an inherently error prone process. Quality scores of variant calling results in NGS studies is a key utility for identifying and prioritizing variants for validation in clinical practice. We investigated the robustness of a wide range of quality scores using bootstrap resampling of the short reads resulting from an NGS exome sequencing study, and evaluated their use as additional quality scores to characterize the called variants. Besides quality scores from the measurement process itself and the biological and clinical relevance of a variant, the bootstrap derived quality scores provide an additional information source for validation prioritization. Additionally, our results indicate possibilities for decreasing the depth of the NGS measurement and increasing the robustness of bioinformatic post-processing.**

Keywords— **NGS, Bioinformatics, Bootstrap, Robustness, Variant Calling, Quality Scores**

I. Introduction

Despite the increasing prevalence of access to next-generation sequencing systems, some of the fundamental issues regarding the robustness of results have yet to be fully addressed [1].

Next generation sequencing commonly follows a workflow that consists of five basic steps;

1. Sample preparation and sequencing: target DNA is isolated and amplified according to the protocol specified by the NGS platform vendor. The resulting reads of several hundred base pairs in length are assigned per-base quality scores. The de facto industry standard measure for base quality is the Phred [2] score, which is the log 10 probability of a single base call being incorrect.
2. Read alignment or assembly; if the target DNA sequence is known, then the reads are aligned to the reference sequence. In case of de novo DNA sequencing, the reads are assembled into contiguous consensus strands.
3. Variant calling: all the reads that map to each location in the target region are evaluated to identify any difference from the reference sequence.
4. Validation: validation is key in clinical settings, and it requires confirmation of both positive and negative results [3,4].
5. Result interpretation: the results of the measurement are used in clinical decision support or are analyzed for functional effects in studies

In this paper we wish to address the common issue of the uncertainty of variant calling. Due to the large amounts of measurement data generated during a sequencing run, it can be difficult to distinguish variants that are called purely as a result of low coverage and the accumulation of random errors or as a result of a platform or sequence specific errors.

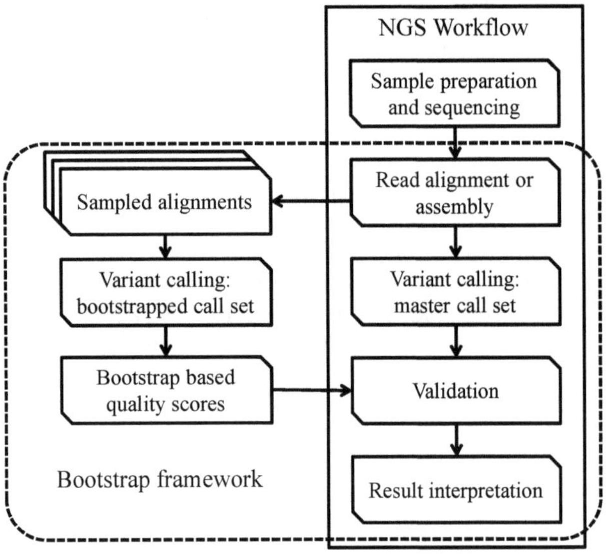

Fig. 1 High-level overview of the NGS workflow and of the bootstrap framework, where a set of alignments are sampled from the master alignment, with variant calling performed also on the sampled alignments. The bootstrap method is used to calculate additional quality metrics and the models trained from the bootstrapped data is used to prioritize variants for validation.

Our hypothesis is that performing bootstrapping on the alignments produced from a sequencing run can provide us with valuable additional information regarding the validity and reliability of results (Fig. 1.). This robustness information can be used to prioritize variants for validation in clinical practice.

Á. Jobbágy (ed.), *First European Biomedical Engineering Conference for Young Investigators*,
IFMBE Proceedings 50, DOI: 10.1007/978-981-287-573-0_11

II. MATERIALS AND METHODS

For this study we chose the exonic regions of chromosome 1 from the genome of Coriell NA12878 [5] as our master dataset. Exome sequencing was performed by the NIST Genome in a Bottle Consortium [6] via amplification with the Nextera Rapid Exome Capture kit, on an Illumina HiSeq 2500 platform at an average coverage depth of 50 (Fig. 2.). We used the Illumina Platinum Genomes reference calls sets as our validation dataset, which was sequenced using the TruSeq DNA PCR-Free Library Prep Kit and sequenced at 50x coverage on an Illumina HiSeq 2000 platform [7]. This particular sample has been a target of many sequencing studies since the early development of NGS.

Short read alignment was performed with the Burrows-Wheeler Aligner (BWA) [8].

Variant calling was performed with a well-established variant caller; the Unified Genotyper tool, which is a part of the Broad Institute's Genome Analysis Toolkit (GATK) [9,10,11]. For a comparison of the sensitivity and specificity of variant calling software, see [12]. Identical default settings were used to perform the variant calling on the master dataset, as well as on the bootstrapped datasets.

The validation dataset contained a total of 3268 calls where the genome of the subject differed from the human reference genome (HG19). Variant calling of the master alignment resulted in 3191 calls. Comparing the validation and the master call set reveals that there are 361 false negatives and 284 false positives in the master call set. Of the 361 false negatives, 120 were found in the bootstrapped results. The bootstrapped results also contained 3780 true negative variants that were not called in either the validation or the master call set. Table 1. shows the results of all the aggregated calls in the bootstrapped dataset.

Source	Status	Count	Marker
In validation and master	True positive	2907	■
In master only	False positive	284	▲
In validation and bootstrap	False negative	120	◆
Only in bootstrap	True negative	3780	●
Only in validation	Missed	241	

Table 1 Counts of each variant call type and their corresponding categories. Marker types note the designations used in the results section.

When performing bootstrapping, we are typically trying to determine a feature of objects given an unknown distribution[13]. Since the distribution P is unknown, we will use

$$\overline{x} = \{x_1, \ldots x_n\} \sim P \qquad (1)$$

to estimate the feature. We also have to estimate the goodness of our estimate, by calculating the variance of our estimate. We resample our x input data into B separate x_i^* bootstrap samples, where the size of x_i^* is identical to $\overline{x}$, and it is drawn from a uniform distribution of $\overline{x}$.

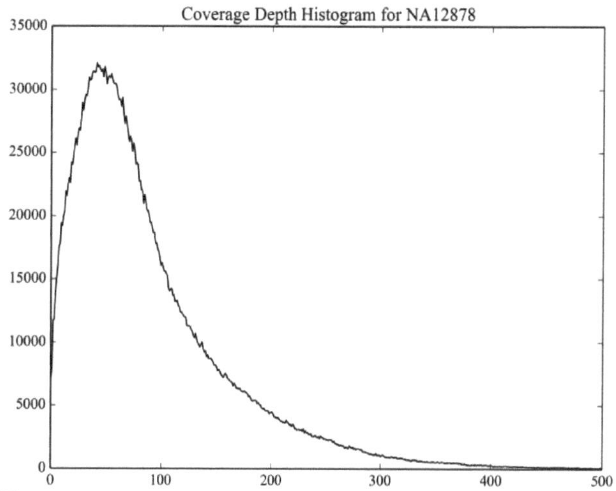

Fig. 2 The average coverage for the exonic regions of chromosome 1 is above 50x. The X axis represents the coverage depths, and the Y axis shows depth counts.

To examine the variance of an arbitrary *s(.)* statistic, we calculate it for each resampled dataset. The bootstrap estimation of the standard error for a *s(.)* can be calculated as follows:

$$se_{boot} = \sqrt{\sum_{i=1}^{B} \frac{(s(x_i^*) - \overline{s})^2}{B-1}} \qquad (2)$$

where $\overline{s}$ is the spread of the statistic above all bootstrapped samples (3).

$$\overline{s} = \sum_{i=1}^{B} s(x_i^*) / B \qquad (3)$$

We resampled the master alignment 100 times to produce the bootstrapped inputs for the variant caller, and then aggregated the results by aggregating the quality parameters for identical call sites, and calculated the bootstrapped standard error for each quality parameter.

The following quality parameters were examined in this study:

QUAL: Overall call quality score assigned to a call by the Unified Genotyper.

DP: Approximate read depth at the call site, low quality alignments are filtered out.

GQ: Genotype quality score, Phred-scaled.

SOR: Symmetric Odds Ratio of a 2x2 contingency table to detect strand bias.

FS: Phred-scaled p-value using Fisher's exact test to detect strand bias.

The standard error of the above parameters was calculated, along with the relative standard error *RSE* as per (4).

$$RSE = \frac{se_{boot}}{E(s(\overline{x}^{*}))} \quad (4)$$

III. Results

Principal component analysis of the initial 5 quality parameters and the total of 5+10 calculated parameters revealed that initially 3 factors were needed to capture 90% of the variance, while 6 factors were needed from the calculated dataset to capture at the same level, thus determining whether the standard error estimates contained significantly more information than the quality values alone.

We trained binary logistic regression classifiers using SPSS v17 [14] to compare the true positive results against false positives and false negatives. The forward stepwise method with Wald setting was used in model construction to select variables. The probability threshold was 0.05 for entering a variable into the model, and was 0.1 for removing a variable from the model. Preliminary results indicate that the bootstrap-based quality scores are informative as many of them are entered into the models. Sensitivity was increased from 96.2% to 97.5%, and specificity increased from 91.5% to 92.9% (for models, see Table 2).

Our models demonstrate that false positive and false negative results can be distinguished based on our quality scores (Fig. 3). Each marker represents a variant call, where green squares are true positives, blue diamonds are false negatives, red triangles are false positives, black circles are true negatives.

Plotting the relative standard error of the SOR score on the X axis with the log QUAL score on the Y axis shows that false negative results unearthed through bootstrapping have low quality scores (Fig. 3.A).

Plotting the relative standard error of the SOR score on the X axis and the log QUAL score on the Y axis shows that false positive and false negative calls are well separated from true negative calls (Fig. 3.B).

Plotting the relative standard error of the quality score on the X axis with the $\log_{10}$ coverage depth of each variant on the Y axis shows that false positive and false negative calls are often found in areas of high coverage, and are indicated by their high relative standard errors (Fig. 3.C).

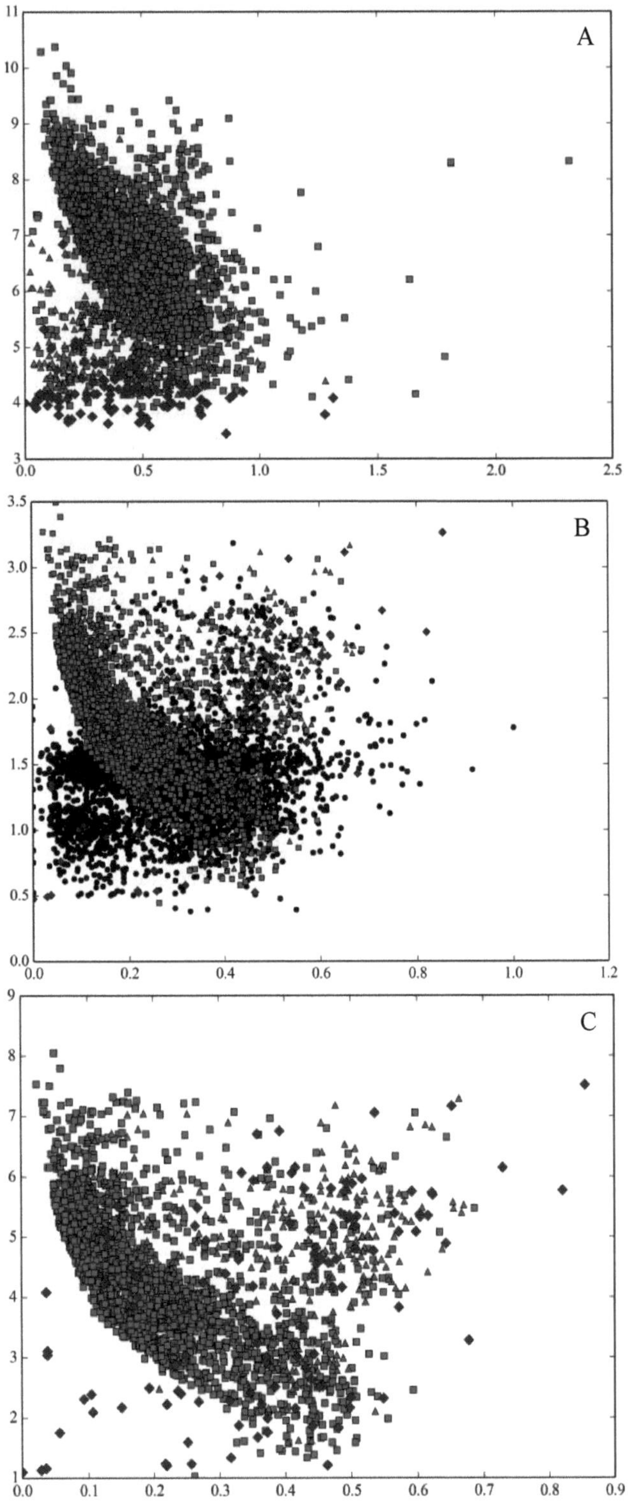

Fig. 3 Visualization of quality parameters which show marked correlation with variant call status.

Table 2 Binary logistic regression models for separating true positives from false negatives and from false positives.

Original quality scores only			
True positive/false negative		True positive/false positive	
Variable	Exp(B)	Variable	Exp(B)
QUAL	1.007	QUAL	1.002
DP	0.997	DP	0.997
SOR	0.822	GQ	0.982
Constant	3.077	SOR	0.622
		FS	0.971
		Constant	44.108
Percentage correct:	96.2%	Percentage correct:	91.5%

With bootstrapped standard errors and relative standard errors			
True positive/false negative		True positive/false positive	
Variable	Exp(B)	Variable	Exp(B)
QUAL	1.001	QUAL	1.001
se_{boot} GQ	0.906	se_{boot} GQ	0.919
se_{boot} FS	0.913	se_{boot} FS	0.889
RSE QUAL	0.004	RSE QUAL	0.001
RSE DP	2.40E+04	RSE DP	5.85E+05
RSE SOR	59.673	RSE SOR	52.941
Constant	1.648	Constant	3.925
Percentage correct:	97.5%	Percentage correct:	92.9%

IV. CONCLUSIONS

The alignment and variant calling in the post-processing of next-generation sequencing data is a complex, context-sensitive step around a variant. Both in research and clinical practice, the validation of called variants is still a necessary step, which is guided by quality scores from the measurement process itself and multitudes of biological, clinical properties (annotations) of a variant. Bootstrapping provides us with further information about the robustness of variant calling based on a solid mathematical framework . Our preliminary results show us that relative standard error of key quality parameters indicates that a variant call requires further investigation or validation, especially in cases where there is ample coverage.

V. FUTURE WORK

A systematic statistical evaluation of the predictive power of bootstrap-based quality scores is a necessary step, also investigating the use of earlier quality scores from the measurement process itself, the parameterization of bioinformatics tools and the size and number of samples tested.. Note that the improved performance of discrimination models hints at the possibility of decreasing the depth of the NGS measurement, while keeping the performance level, i.e. a trade-off between molecular measurement and computation. We plan to characterize this relation quantitatively.

ACKNOWLEDGMENT

The publication was supported by the OTKA 109268 project, and by the János Bolyai Research Scholarship of the Hungarian Academy of Sciences (P. Antal).

CONFLICT OF INTEREST

The authors declare that they have no conflict of interest.

REFERENCES

1. Gargis AS, Kalman L, Berry MW, Bick DP, Dimmock DP, Hambuch T, Lu F, Lyon E, Voelkerding KV, Zehnbauer BA et al (2012) Assuring the quality of next-generation sequencing in clinical laboratory practice. Nature Biotechnology 30:1033-1036.
2. Ewing B, Green P (1998). Base-calling of automated sequencer traces using phred. II. Error probabilities. Genome Res. 8 (3): 186–194. DOI 10.1101/gr.8.3.186.
3. Rehm HL, Bale SJ, Bayrak-Toydemir P, Berg JS, Brown KK, Deignan JL, Friez MJ, Funke BH, Hegde MR, Lyon E et al (2013) ACMG clinical laboratory standards for next-generation sequencing. Genetics in Medicine 15:733-747.
4. Lubin IMK, Lisa, Gargis AS (2013) Guidelines and Approaches to Compliance with Regulatory and Clinical Standards: Quality Control Procedures and Quality Assurance Next Generation Sequencing 2013:255-273.
5. McVean et Al (2012) An integrated map of genetic variation from 1,092 human genomes. Nature 491, 56–65 DOI 10.1038/nature11632
6. Genome in a Bottle consortium https://sites.stanford.edu/abms/giab
7. Illumina Platinum Genomes at http://www.illumina.com/platinumgenomes/
8. Li H, and Durbin R (2009) Fast and accurate short read alignment with Burrows-Wheeler Transform. Bioinformatics, 25:1754-60.
9. McKenna A, Hanna M, Banks E et al (2010) The Genome Analysis Toolkit. Genome Research 20:1297-303
10. DePristo M, Banks E, Poplin R (2011) A framework for variation discovery and genotyping using next-generation DNA sequencing data. Nature Genetics 43:491-498
11. Van der Auwera GA, Carneiro M, Hartl C (2013) From FastQ Data to High-Confidence Variant Calls. Current Protocols in Bioinformatics 43:11.10.1-11.10.33
12. Yi M, Zhao Y, Jia L, He M, Kebebew E, Stephens RM, (2014) Performance comparison of SNP detection tools with illumina exome sequencing data. Nucleic Acids Research 2014;42(12):e101. DOI 10.1093/nar/gku392
13. Efron B, Tibshirani RJ (1993) An Introduction to the Bootstrap. Chapman & Hall
14. SPSS Inc. Released 2008. SPSS 17.0. Chicago: SPSS Inc.

Author: Peter Sarkozy
Institute: Budapest University of Technology and Economics, Department of Measurement and Information Systems
Street: Magyar tudósok körútja 2.
City: Budapest
Country: Hungary
Email: psarkozy@mit.bme.hu

Web-Pacs in Imaging Medical: A Teaching and Visualization Tool in Clinical Trial

M.L. Mora[1], B.A. Prado[1], C.I. Salazar[2], J.E. Restrepo[1], and J.I. Garcia[3]

[1] Cooperativa de Colombia University/ School of Engineering and School Psychology Neuro-Spin Laboratory, Cali - Colombia
[2] Cauca University / School of Humanities, Popayan - Colombia
[3] Valle University / School Mechanical Engineering Laboratory, Cali - Colombia

Abstract —This paper presents Information systems that have advances in clinical centers of medical image diagnosis. The information in clinical trial the image medical is very important. PACS (picture archiving and communication system) is an evolving healthcare technology for the short and long term storage, retrieval, management, distribution and presentation of medical images. Our main aim is to provide a new teaching and visualization tool for supporting clinical Web-Pacs involving different hospital and research center institutions. These clinical information systems are oriented to individual patient information management, but not to group management with different experimental conditions. The Web Pacs systems manage patient groups, but not available research more accurate of algorithms that help the image processing development that benefit the research. Investigation of diseases in different applications as: new clinical studies in psychiatry, neurology, cardiology and oncology. New needs for storing images arise from the analysis of the same images, with this we made massive load of images that are analyzed with high-performance algorithms. To perform the mass storage of images that can be analyzed with algorithms at high performance we create a new model of Web-Pacs a teaching and visualization tool in clinical trial. This model contains a cluster distribution that performs research in image processing with its object of investigation. The distribution of model Web – Pac's is presented below with your research cluster in model visualization tool in Clinical Trial Neuro – Spin Laboratory.

Keywords— **PACS (picture archiving and communication system), Psychiatry, Neurology, Cardiology, Oncology, Algorithms. Clinical Trial and cluster.**

I. Introduction

Healthcare and Medical Imaging in particular, are undergoing significant change as they adapt and evolve to cope with society's current and future healthcare needs. Health Information Technology (IT) and medical devices are well known by radiologists, who have witnessed tremendous growth and advances in both. The technology for acquiring, storing, retrieving, displaying, and distributing images has advanced dramatically in recent years.

The system in imaging radiology as: cardiology, neurology, oncology are seamlessly linked with information. A picture archiving and communication system (PACS) [1] is a medical imaging technology which provides economical storage and convenient access to images from multiple modalities (source machine types).

Electronic images and reports are transmitted digitally via PACS; this eliminates the need to manually file, retrieve, or transport film jackets. The imaging modalities such as X-ray plain film (PF), computed tomography (CT) [2] and magnetic resonance imaging (MRI), network for the transmission of patient information, workstations for interpreting and reviewing images, and archives for the storage and retrieval of images and reports.

Combined with available and emerging web technology, PACS has the ability to deliver timely and efficient access to images, interpretations, and related data. PACS breaks down the physical and time barriers associated with traditional film-based image retrieval, distribution, and display. New needs arise in medical image management that exceed the capabilities hospital information system PACS. To store this type of information in records of medical image, we use cluster of investigation in Clinical Trial [3] the laboratories for the analysis of medical image.

This paper is organized as following. In Section II, Structure of the Model is presented. Section III shows the processes with images in cluster of investigation. At last, in Section IV Conclusion, Acknowledgment and References.

II. Structure of the Model

We describe one model. This one is a detailed description of all the technical tasks related with the acquisition and processing of medical and other components. Research in hospitals units, universities, or in the pharmaceutical industry and Centers of investigation. This model of clusters has his application for Neuro - Spin Laboratory at the Cooperative de Colombia University South America. Pioneering laboratory in the processing image with cluster of investigation. The cluster of investigation used in the paper

Á. Jobbágy (ed.), *First European Biomedical Engineering Conference for Young Investigators*,
IFMBE Proceedings 50, DOI: 10.1007/978-981-287-573-0_12

is summarized in the Table 1. In summary a set of cluster procedure is implemented in laboratory as clinical trial, as described:

1. Cluster Definition Protocols: lines the investigation are acquired in different modalities by scanner medical system.

2. Cluster in Image Processing: this module applies technique in diagnostic medicine. In the last years the radiological sciences have highly expanded in different modalities; CT (Computed Tomography) Positron Emission (PET), DTI (image Tensor Diffusion) [10] and other techniques. The appearance new scanner of Magnetic Resonance Image (MRI), make possible the reconstruction the image and processing and data analysis are development model mathematical algorithms [4].

3. Cluster in Diagnosis detection: the image volumetric is analyzed with SPM Statistical Parametric Mapping, the volumetric content DICOM is converted to format *.img, this format is computerized for processing the algorithms Mathematicians.

4. Cluster Reconstruction and Restoration Image: This Digital image reconstruction is a robust means by which the underlying images hidden in blurry and noisy data can be revealed. The main challenge is sensitivity to measurement noise in the input data, which can be magnified strongly, resulting in large artifacts in the reconstructed image [5].

5. Cluster Registration Image: Using registration we can compare and integrate the data obtained from different measurements [6].

6. Cluster Quantification Model: are obtained according to mathematical and physical models providing data on image processing, we first quantify the algorithm of definition to measure diseases.

7. Cluster Computational Biology: biological images are analyzing and utilizing. Images with big data in DNA's sequence and bases data biological.

8. Cluster Graphical Computation: Development image study of 3D-dimensional computer graphics, it also encompasses 2D-dimensional graphics and image processing [7].

9. Cluster Virtual Reality: The module in virtual reality involves the development and combination of areas such as collision handling, haptic rendering, physical simulation, and volumetric visualization. The simulator's input data comes from computed-tomography and magnetic-resonance-imaging images and other modalities in images of the patients [8].

10. Cluster Development Software: Many software of development are programmed for applications in medical image, these applications as: Slicer 3D developed by Harvard Medical School, it is possible to realize measures and calculations of algorithms applied to software in medical image [9].

11. Cluster Process Simulation: The logistic calculation of estimation allows to recognized form of organization and estimation the series the time [10] in processes. The locations in time of series and other applications of mathematical order, to contribute a process in the organization information. Optimization the data in compression of Image. Also this cluster develops biomedical instrumentation in simulation and the construction of protocol clinic in rehabilitation.

The cluster of investigation implemented, It refers to the following modules as: Image Processing, Different modalities of image are analyzed MRI – DTI (Magnetic Resonance Imaging – Diffusion Tensor Imaging), CT (Computed Tomography), Positron Emission (PET). Module de Detection the image, this one of analyzes the image with software SPM Statistical Parametric Mapping). Cluster Reconstruction and Restoration Image, this A Bayesian interpretation of the regularization techniques is given which clarifies the role of the tuning parameters and indicates how they could be estimated the image. Module Registration Image, we are concerned with the segmentation of structures within the brain particularly the cerebral cortex, but also subcortical structures from volumetric T1 – weighted MRI images. Module Quantification Model; this one develops the algorithm's in mathematical base with the result of the processes applied in the different clusters of investigation. The processing development in Graphical Computation and reality virtual it is possible in reconstruction the image. For this development we apply software in engineering.

Table 1. Clusters of investigation

Cluster	Position	Area Research
Definition Protocol	1	Biomedicine
Image Processing	2	Biomedicine
Diagnosis detection	3	Biomedicine
Reconstruction and Restoration	4	Biomedicine
Registration Image	5	Biomedicine
Quantification Model	6	Engineering
Computational Biology	7	Biomedicine
Graphical Computation	8	Engineering
Virtual Reality	9	Engineering
Development Software	10	Engineering
Process Simulation	11	Engineering

In Fig.1, show clusters Neuro-Spin Laboratory in clinical trial the research. This figure shows the cluster for module of investigation. Our application of research are Biomedicine and Engineering, it is possibility for progress in human.

We study diseases in application medical, with different pathologies as: neurology, oncology, biology, psychiatric, radiology all in techniques the Image Medical.

Medical Image analysis provides new results in the field of medical and biological image analysis, with special emphasis on efforts related to the applications of computer vision, virtual reality and robotics to biomedical imaging.

The clusters in laboratory contribute to the basic science of processing, analyzing and utilizing medical and biological images for these purposes. The Clusters are interested in approaches that utilize biomedical image datasets at all spatial scales, ranging from molecular cellular imaging to tissue/organ imaging.

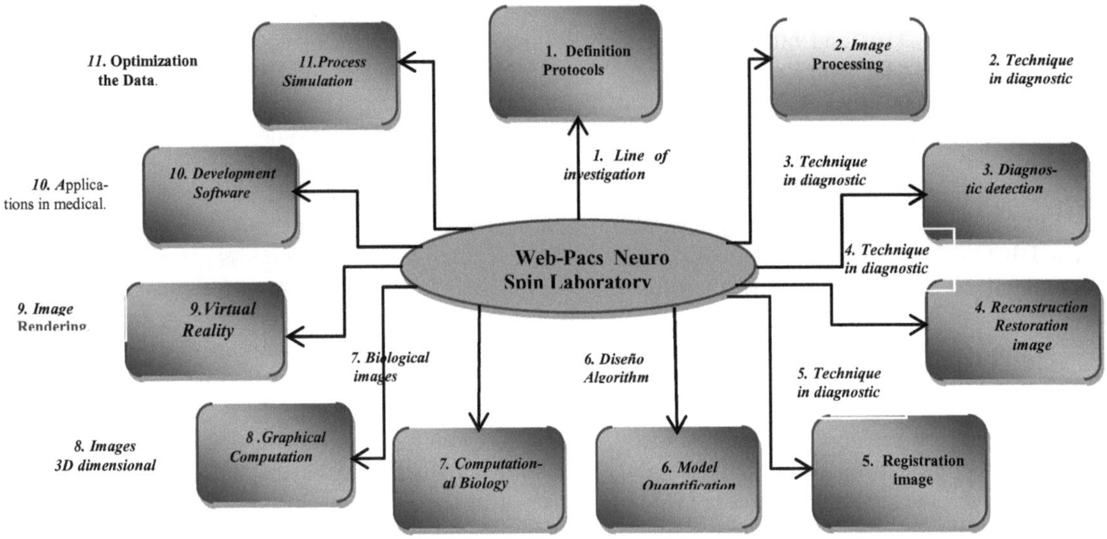

Fig. 1 Clusters Neuro Spin Lababoratory

Our laboratory development and implementation of algorithms in clusters research, strategies based on the use of various models (geometrical, statistical, physical, functional, etc.) to solve the following types of problems, using biomedical image datasets: representation of pictorial data, visualization, feature extraction, segmentation, inter-study and inter-subject registration, longitudinal, temporal studies, image – guided surgery and intervention, texture, shape and motion measurements, spectral analysis, digital anatomical atlases, statistical shape analysis, computational anatomy (modelling normal anatomy and its variations), computational physiology (modelling organs and living systems for image analysis, simulation and training), virtual and augmented reality for therapy planning and guidance, telemedicine with medical images, telepresence in medicine, telesurgery and image-guided medical robots, etc.

III. METHODOLOGY.

A. ***The Implementation structure of clusters***. As can be seen in Fig. 1. The implementation involves eleven (11) different steps. Our next goal is to create a user friendly framework for visualizing the different modalities image and processing. A further objective is to preserve the spatial representation of the anatomical regions of interest and to integrate this information with knowledge about the relations among anatomical structures.

Accordingly, we wanted to create a labelling system for each of the anatomical structures that was based on hierarchical relations. Patients Identifying information, including patients' names, initials, or hospital numbers, should not be published in written descriptions, pathologic, and information is essential for scientific purposes in medical Imaging

B. ***The clusters in image Description***. Diagnosis detection, reconstruction, restoration and segmentation image, allows developing algorithms. Image registration is a process in which final information is gained from different data sources. Image restoration is based on mathematical or probabilistic models of image degradation. Image segmentation means to partition an input image into its constituent parts or objects identifying a region of interest (ROI).

C. **Transform model estimation:** Identifying details the mathematical model in image. This parameter the MR images of the scanned in brain is made with a set N slices and each slice is extracted from a three dimensional (3D) gradient echo (SPGR) acquisition (Using $= 30° \mid TR = 20$, $TE = 5$). Each image is represented, in a computational grid which discretize the image domain ($\gamma \epsilon R^2$), by (n x m) Shanon[11]. Others models the transformation can be:

(DWT) Discrete Wavelet Transform, Fourier Transform FT). matrix, where **n** is the number of nodes along the width and **m** is the number of nodes along the height of the slices. The matrix coefficients represents the grey level intensity at each pixel ($X_i, Y_j \in (\gamma \epsilon R^2)$, $i = 1..n$, $j = 1 \ldots m$) . The a simple method - algorithm that develops the correction image, this correction method that avoids the problems of intensity artifacts in MR images. This method is based on the theory of **PDE** (Equations differential Partial) and uses a multiscale low – pass filter based on a Gaussian Kernel to extract the artifact. All this theory makes possible the correction an image applying mathematical model the **PDE.**

IV. CONCLUSIONS

In This paper a clusters structure of research is implemented with application in Biomedical and Engineering. In this methods was implemented 3 steps where integrated research clusters. The goal in the first step is create user friendly framework for visualization the different modalities image, where medical image analysis provides new results in the field of medical and biological image analysis, with applications of computer vision, virtual reality and robotics to biomedical imaging.

In the step 2, procedures for the image processing as registration, restoration, reconstruction and segmentation are implemented. These processes will be made in cases where the required image and the result can be an algorithm structure.

In the step 3, A mathematical model is created for transform model estimation in the image. The parameter the MR images of the scanned in brain is made with a set N slices and each slice is extracted from a three dimensional (3D). These data are processed in computational model mathematical as Theory Shanon in PDE (Equations differential Partial) and other authors. Models the transformation can.

ACKNOWLEDGMENT

Acknowledgment and References, the Institutions scientific School Medicine Harvard (HMS) Psychiatry Neuroimaging Laboratory Dr. Martha Shenton, MA -U.S.A., Research Institute Neuro -Psychiatry Lopez Ibor Dr. Juan J. Lopez Ibor and Clinical hospital San Carlos department of diagnosis for image, Dr. Juan Arrazola in Madrid - Spain, with contribution in image medicates and in measurements that are applied in different pathologies.

REFERENCES

1. Majkowski G.E., (2003) Fault tolerant database for picture archiving and communication systems. Patents US6564336 B1 General Electric Company.
2. Depeursinge Adrien, Kurtz Camille, F. Christopher. Beaulieu, Sandy, Rubin Daniel, Rubin Daniel. (2014) Predicting Visual Semantic Descriptive Terms from Radiological Image Data: Preliminary Results with Liver Lesions in CT. DOI 10.1109/TMI.2014.2321347, IEEE Transactions on Medical Imaging.
3. Hernández J.A., Acuña J. Cesar, Castro Ma. Valeria, Marcos E., et al (2007) Web – PACS for Multicenter Clinical Trials. IEEE Transactions On Information Technology in Biomedicine vol.11 No.1: 87–93.
4. Hernández J.A., Mora Martha L., Emanuele Schiavi., Pablo Toharia. (2004) Rf Inhomogeneity Correction Algorithm in Magnetic Resonance Imaging. Biological and Medical Data Analysis – Spring Verlang.
5. R.C. Puetter, T.R.Gosnell, Amos Yahil (2005) Digital Image Reconstruction: Deblurring and Denoising. Annual Review of Astronomy and Astrophysics. Vol. 43: 139-194 (Volumen publication date August 2005) DOI: 10.1146/annurev.astro.43.112904.104850.
6. Singla Jimmy (2012) Technique of image Registration in digital Image Processing. International Journal of Information Technology and Knowledge Management July – December 2012, Volumen 5, No. 2 pp 239-243.
7. Shellshear Evan, Ytterlid Rubin (2014) Fast Distance Queries for Triangles, Lines and Points Using SSE Instructions. Journal of Computer Graphics Techniques Vol.3 No. 4 pag. 86 -110.
8. Echegaray G., Herrera I., Aguinaga I, Buchart C. Borro D. (2014) A Brain Surgery Simulator, IEEE computer Graphics and Applications. Vol. 34, No.3, pp. 12-18, May-June.
9. Mahmood N. H., Yong C.Y.,Chew K.M., Arifin I., Image Processing Software Package in Medical Imaging. (2012) International Journal of Computational engineering Research ISSN: 2250-3005.
10. Kirchgassner G., Wolters J., Hassler U. (2013) Introduction to Modern Time Series Analysis. Springer Text in Business and Economics ISBN: 978-3-642-33435-1.
11. G. Sapiro. Geometric partial differential equations and image analysis. ISBN 0-521-79075-1 (2006) Cambridge University Press.

Assisting Humans with Special Needs: Curriculum for HUman-TOol Interaction Network - HUTON

N. Jorgovanović, D.J. Đozić, D. Bojanić, V. Ilić, and Ž. Tepić

Department for Systems, Signals and Control, Faculty of Technical Sciences, University of Novi Sad, Serbia

Abstract— **The arising field of biomedical engineering is becoming more popular worldwide. TEMPUS project "Assisting humans with special needs: Curriculum for HUman-TOol interaction Network - HUTON" has a goal to provide new curriculum and necessary equipment for three universities in Serbia, as well as to establish a collaboration between nine partners involved in project from four countries (Serbia, Slovenia, Greece and Italy) for future research in the field of mechatronic in medical rehabilitation. This is of great importance for institutions in Serbia to be recognized and introduced to EU scientific community.**

Keywords—**Study programme, Rehabilitation, Mechatronic, TEMPUS.**

I. Introduction

The use of computers, robotics and/or other equipment has become practically a part of every field, including healthcare. Biomedical engineering is becoming more popular, and is in great expansion worldwide. TEMPUS project is one of many projects financed by EU which goal is to consolidate and unify EU and non EU countries in the research program and by that way make a network of experts which will work together and give better contribution to science. This TEMPUS project "Assisting humans with special needs: Curriculum for HUman-TOol interaction Network - HUTON" [1] has a goal to provide an interdisciplinary curriculum as well as provide necessary equipment which will be used at universities and other institutions in Serbia involved in this project, in order to train and gain experts in the domain of mechatronics, rehabilitation and medicine. By this way Republic of Serbia will get more involved in the research in the field of Biomedical Engineering and give its contribution to world's science community.

II. Project

TEMPUS project "Assisting humans with special needs: Curriculum for HUman-TOol interaction Network - HUTON" is developing the interdisciplinary and multidisciplinary curriculum and the training network for the optimized use of technology that improves quality of life of humans with special needs with the following specific objectives:

a) development of the new interdisciplinary and multidisciplinary accredited curriculum leading to the master degree in the domain of technologies for humans with special needs,
b) setup of the training network in Republic of Serbia in the domain of mechatronics, rehabilitation engineering and medicine, and neurorehabilitation that enables the delivery of the new interdisciplinary and multidisciplinary curriculum, and
c) training of staff for providing on-the-job education and new employment opportunities, and hence providing better medical services for humans with special needs.

Project includes nine partners from four countries: University of Belgrade, Serbia (coordinator); University of Novi Sad, Serbia; Sate University of Novi Pazar, Serbia; University of Patras, Greece; University of Genoa, Italy; University of Ljubljana, Slovenia; Clinic for rehabilitation "Dr Miroslav Zotović", Belgrade, Serbia; Child and Youth Health Care Institute of Vojvodina, Novi Sad, Serbia; and Special Hospital for treatment of Neuromuscular Diseases, Novi Pazar, Serbia.

The purpose of this curriculum is to:

a) contribute to development of modern and efficient healthcare system which is based on modern education programs and the use of new medical technologies, and
b) enable integration of modern information technologies in medicine system in order to enhance the quality of life for people with special needs.

It should be enhanced that this curriculum gives synergy effects based on interdisciplinary and multidisciplinary approach and provides significant progress in providing services to people with special needs. It is in line with the trend of the education system in Republic of Serbia to develop new forms of sustainable long curricula especially in terms of integration of Serbia into the European family, and implementation of general identified trends that have been validated in Europe.

Direct users of this result are clinical partners in HUTON project, but the program is open to other institutes and medical centers in Republic of Serbia as well.

Á. Jobbágy (ed.), *First European Biomedical Engineering Conference for Young Investigators*,
IFMBE Proceedings 50, DOI: 10.1007/978-981-287-573-0_13

A. Curriculum

The curriculum is modeled based on programs in other developed countries in Europe (Germany, Netherlands, Greece, etc.) where system is proven to give good results ([1, 2, 3]). It is based on hands-on approach and project based learning, in which students are encouraged to learn through practical work, real, interesting and state of the art projects. Students will work in clinical environment as well as in laboratories by which they will obtain important and necessary experience and knowledge for an excellent future expert. New mechatronic systems will be set in the clinics where staff will be educated for their optimal use.

The HUTON graduates will be prepared to think analytically and creatively, examine issues from a wide variety of perspectives, identify problems and employ appropriate strategies for rehabilitation, evaluate and apply information needed to solve a problem, and use scientific methods of inquiry.

The curriculum is composed of four mandatory and eleven elective courses which enable students to focus and expand their knowledge in fields of their interest.

Mandatory courses:

- Mechatronics Systems
- Principles of Motor Control in Humans
- Disability Assessment Methods
- Signals and Systems in Rehabilitation

Elective courses:

- External Control of Biological Actuators
- Mechanics of Robots
- Rehabilitation Systems Control
- Pneumatic and Hydraulic Actuators
- Electrical and Magnetic Actuators Sensors for Mechatronics System
- Methods and Instrumentation for Motor Measurement
- Microcomputers
- Scientific Research in Rehabilitation
- Robotics in Rehabilitation
- Biostatistics

III. EQUIPMENT

Project HUTON includes procurement of necessary mechatronic equipment which will be equally distributed to all institutions that are partners of the project and are in Republic of Serbia. In order for courses in curriculum to be better prepared, and students better understand the concept, specific equipment was needed to be purchased that would meet curriculum's needs. We have chosen equipment in such way to cover as much spheres of rehabilitation as possible and in the same way fit in the budget. By this way students can get specific knowledge of all necessary parts of rehabilitation. Some of mechatronic rehabilitation systems to be used for the teaching are shown and presented below.

A. Robotic assistant for upper extremities is a workstation for clinical use

The workstation (Figure 1) allows a range of exercise games with adjustable difficulty levels and a standardized hand and arm function tests. The workstation includes:

a) standardized upper limb exercises representing activities of daily life (ADL),
b) intensive training with motivating games,
c) tracing of functional improvements with an automated, objective hand and arm function tests and
d) possibility for therapists to tele-supervise clients from anywhere.

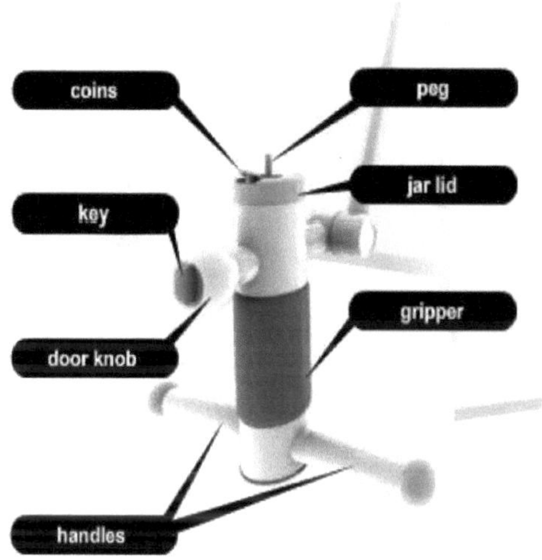

Figure 1 Workstation for exercise for upper extremities

B. Robotic assistant for lower extremities rehabilitation

The robot assistant for lower extremities is a motorized, body support system which secures a patient from falling and reduces a physical stress to therapists (Figure 2). The system includes ground level hands-free walking indoors/outdoors (flat terrain), walking speed regulation from 0m/s to 1.2 m/s, adjustable support from partly to full body weight support by means of body contour harm, remote control of speed and walking direction, complete power supply independence (battery driven).

C. Movement assessment system

The system for movement assessment helps people with special needs to gain insight into their movement (gait)

(Figure 3). It includes a set of small size and light weight sensors units, battery operated sensors units with 3D accelerometers and 3D gyroscopes, wireless communication of each unit with a host computer and a USB receiver.

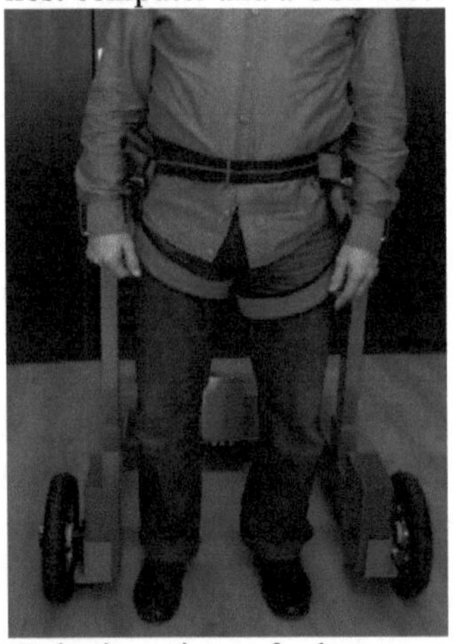

Figure 2 Robotic assistant for lower extremities

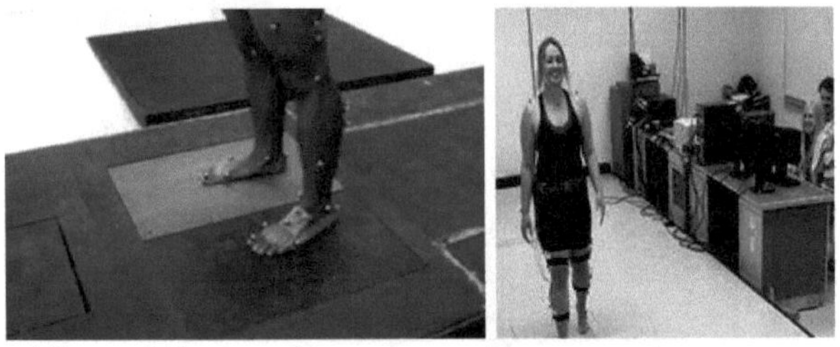

Figure 3 System for movement assessment - sensors mounted on human

D. Ground reaction force assessment system

The system for ground reaction force assessment (Figure 4) is used to record and analyze ground force that patients are making during gait and use it during their rehabilitation process. System includes insole type sensors allowing analysis of ground reaction force distribution, size adjustment mechanism, battery operated sensors, wireless communication with a host computer, USB receiver, and software.

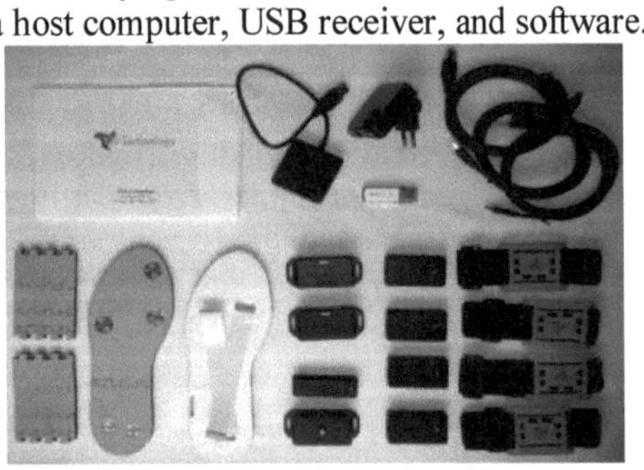

Figure 4 System for ground reaction force assessment

E. Muscle stimulator

The stimulator provides 4 independent channels, recording of EMG signals, setup of stimulation parameters: amplitude up to 100 mA, increment 1mA or less, frequency 1-150Hz, pulse width 30-400 us, and it is battery powered.

F. Biofeedback system

The system allows mental and physical exercise feedback used for a training of the brain. The feedback system includes the recording capabilities of electrophysiological signals originating from brain and muscles. It also provides visual/auditive/somatosensory and other modalities of interfacing with a trainee.

The system includes multichannel amplifier for cortical and muscle signals, interface to a PC/smart phone/other and the appropriate display, software for real-time processing and selection of gaming based scenarios for feedback (Figure 5).

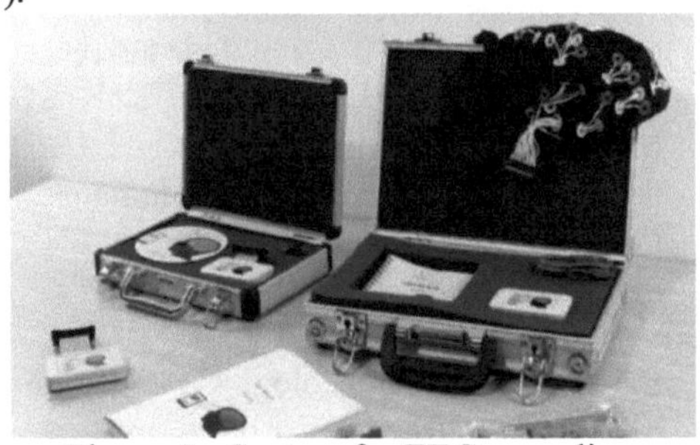

Figure 5 - System for EEG recording

IV. CONCLUSIONS

HUTON project is an EU founded project that is of great value for the education system in Republic of Serbia, as well as for introducing and involving institutes in Serbia in the future scientific EU community. The goal is to provide a new curriculum at three universities in Serbia and connect all nine partners involved in the project from four countries (Serbia, Slovenia, Greece and Italy) into a scientific network with important collaboration for research and training in the field of mehatronic in medical rehabilitation. New curriculum will educate students to the Master degree in the most efficient and proven way (modeled on other EU countries) to becoming experts in the field of mechatronic in medical rehabilitation. Project also includes provision of necessary equipment in order for state of the art research to be done which will have a great impact on the research in Serbia in the arising and popular field of biomedical engineering.

Acknowledgment

We would like to express our gratitude to University of Belgrade as a coordinator, as well as all other universities and clinical institutions that are involved in this TEMPUS project for their engagement and support as well as EU that made this project possible.

References

1. HUTON project website. http://huton.org
2. University of Technology, Eindhoven. https://www.tue.nl/en/education/tue-bachelor-college/undergraduate-programs/biomedical-engineering/study-structure/
3. University of Patras, Greece. http://www.upatras.gr/en/node/134
4. University of Heildelberg, Germany. http://www.uni-heidelberg.de/studium/interesse/faecher/biomed-eng.html

Author: Damir J. Đozić
Institute: Faculty of technical sciences, University of Novi Sad
Street: Trg Dositeja Obradovića 6
City: Novi Sad
Country: Serbia
Email: djozicd@uns.ac.rs

Influence of Ultraviolet and Electron Radiation on Photoelectron Emission Spectra of Lead Sulfide Nanoparticles Embedded in a Matrix of Zirconium Oxide

Yu. Dekhtyar[1], R. Reisfeld[2], M. Romanova[1], T. Saraidarov[2], and I. Surkova[1]

[1] Institute of Biological Engineering and Nanotechnologies, Riga Technical University, Riga, Latvia
[2] Department of Inorganic Chemistry, Hebrew University of Jerusalem, Jerusalem, Israel

Abstract— **Lead sulfide (PbS) nanoparticles embedded in a thin-film matrix of zirconium oxide (ZrO_2), ZrO_2:PbS nanofilms, were studied for application in nanodosimetry of ionizing radiation. Readout of the delivered dose was carried out by measurements of photoelectron emission (PE) current from ZrO_2:PbS nanofilms. PE emission was excited by UV photons having energy of 4.6–6.2 eV. First, the nanofilms were irradiated with non-ionizing UV radiation used as a model of ionizing radiation in order to extract exposure-dependent signal from PE spectra of ZrO_2:PbS nanofilms. It was found that exposure-dependent signal is provided by PbS nanoparticles and it is the decrease of the increment of PE current calculated in energy range of 4.9–5.5 eV. The extracted signal was further analyzed by irradiating ZrO_2:PbS nanofilms with 9 MeV electron radiation. Second degree polynomial relationship was observed between the decrease of the increment of PE spectra calculated in the energy range of 4.9–5.5 eV and dose of electron radiation in the range of 0–10 Gy. Error of dose measurement was calculated for each delivered dose. Error of dose measurement decreases from 65% to 11% when the delivered dose increases from 2 Gy to 5 Gy and doesn't exceed 11% in the dose range of 5–10 Gy. Changes in PE spectra of ZrO_2:PbS nanofilms under influence of electron radiation suggest that the nanofilms have potential to be used in nanodosimetry of ionizing radiation; however, further adjustment of the method is required to reduce dose measurement error.**

Keywords— **lead sulfide, dosimetry, photoelectron emission, ultraviolet radiation, electron radiation.**

I. Introduction

One of the main reasons why ionizing radiation causes biological damage is irreparable rupture of chemical bonds of the DNA molecule. Diameter of the DNA double helix is 2 nm. Field of the dosimetry that studies absorption of dose of radiation in biological nanovolumes is called nanodosimetry. Advances in nanodosimetry will result in deeper understanding of radiobiological effects and increase safety and effectiveness of radiation therapy of cancer. Nanodosimeters which are able to measure dose of ionizing radiation delivered to nanovolumes still do not exist. One of the approaches is to measure number of ionizations caused by radiation in gaseous targets of millimetric dimensions and recalculate the result to the biological nanometric sites using scaling procedure [1]. Another approach is to study thermoluminescent recombination between charge carriers trapped in centers of ~2 nm dimensions under influence of ionizing radiation [2].

This research offers to use nanofilms with embedded nanoparticles as radiation nanodosimeters. The advantage of the nanostructure-based detector is its size which is comparable with nanometric dimensions of the biological targets. This eliminates the error of dose measurement that may be introduced by scaling procedures. Ionizing radiation creates free charge carriers in the material, concentration of those will depend on the delivered dose. In order to store the generated electric charge for a long time, the dosimeter has to be made from semiconductor or dielectric material. In this case free charge carriers (electrons) will move through the conduction band until they are trapped in localized states located inside the band gap. By measuring the number of the trapped electrons, it is possible to evaluate the delivered dose of radiation. This can be done by recording photoelectron emission (PE) excited by ultraviolet (UV) photons having energy of 4–6 eV that is close to work function of the solids. In this case the emitted electrons have kinetic energy of 0.1–1 eV and the emission signal is coming from the depth of 10–100 nm [3,4].

The purpose of this study is to demonstrate the potential application of nanostructures in nanodosimetry of ionizing radiation, providing the readout of the dose by measuring PE from the nanostructures with size similar to DNA molecule. ZrO_2:PbS nanofilms were used which are composed of semiconductor PbS nanoparticles with a diameter of 2.5 nm embedded in a 100 nm thick dielectric matrix of ZrO_2. Lead is a well known absorber of ionizing radiation. ZrO_2 matrix provides physical and chemical stability of PbS nanoparticles.

II. Samples

PbS nanoparticles were embedded in ZrO_2 matrix using sol-gel method described in [5]. The resulting ZrO_2:PbS nanofilms were deposited on the glass substrate.

20% and 50% molar concentration of PbS was used in the experiments. However, ZrO_2 matrix cannot accommo-

Á. Jobbágy (ed.), *First European Biomedical Engineering Conference for Young Investigators*,
IFMBE Proceedings 50, DOI: 10.1007/978-981-287-573-0_14

date more than 30% PbS in a form of nanoparticles [6]. When the molar concentration exceeds 30%, a thin layer of bulk PbS is formed on the surface of ZrO_2. Molar concentration of 50% was used to intensify the PE signal of PbS material in order to distinguish it from the PE signal provided by ZrO_2 matrix.

III. Methods

Two types of radiation were used. At first, ZrO_2:PbS nanofilms with 20% and 50% molar concentration of PbS were irradiated with non-ionizing UV radiation during 0–75 minutes which was used as a model of ionizing radiation. UV light has higher absorption in a shallow depth of the surface compared to other types of electromagnetic radiation; therefore, by using UV, it is easier to observe dose-dependent PE signal of ZrO_2:PbS nanofilms. ZrO_2 matrix was also irradiated as reference. After the extraction of the dose-dependent signal, ZrO_2:PbS nanofilms with 20% molar concentration of PbS were irradiated with 9 MeV electron beam with doses 0–10 Gy and changes of the extracted PE signal were further analyzed.

UV irradiation was carried out using Hamamatsu Photonics Lightningcure LC5 L8222 light source with 200 W mercury-xenon lamp L8251 (250–450 nm, the central wavelength 365 nm). The distance between the output of the light guide and the surface of the samples was 40 cm in order to avoid heating of the samples. UV irradiance at this distance was 5 mW/cm^2.

Electron beam was supplied by medical linear accelerator Clinac 2100C/D Varian. Dose rate was 300 MU/min.

PE current was recorded using a self-made laboratory spectrometer. PE was excited by photons with energy $E = 4.6–6.2$ eV (270–200 nm) generated by deuterium lamp (LOT-Oriel Europe). Emitted electrons were detected using the secondary electron multiplier (SED-6 / ВЭУ-6, Russia) in vacuum $5 \cdot 10^{-5}$ Torr. Detection was made at room temperature. Measurement error of the photon energy was ±0.03 eV in the wavelength range of 200–300 nm.

IV. Results and discussion

A. *Influence of UV radiation*

PE current $N=f(E)$ is a number of emitted electrons per second as a function of the energy of PE exciting photons. PE intensity of ZrO_2:50%PbS nanofilms decreases after UV irradiation and is relatively low after 75 minutes of exposure (Fig. 1).

PE data were fitted to the fifth degree polynomial (coefficient of determination R^2=0.99). In order to characterize influence of UV on concentration of electron emission centers, the derivatives of the PE current in respect to photon energy were taken.

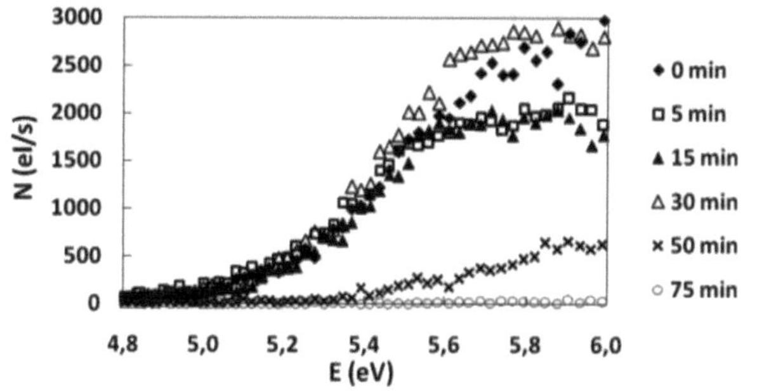

Fig. 1 PE current from ZrO_2:50%PbS nanofilms depending on UV exposure

The derivatives of the non-irradiated ZrO_2:50%PbS nanofilm (Fig. 2) have distinct emission maximum at 5.5 eV with a width from 4.9 to 6.0 eV. The maximum disappears after 50 minutes of UV exposure which means that radiation decreases concentration of the electron emission centers.

For comparison, derivatives of PE spectra of non-irradiated and irradiated ZrO_2 matrix are plotted (Fig. 2). The maxima at 5.5 eV are not observed which means that the emission signal at 4.9–6.0 eV exists due to the presence of PbS nanoparticles in ZrO_2. In addition, ZrO_2 matrix reacts differently to UV radiation than ZrO_2:50%PbS nanofilm, because the intensity of its derivative line increases after irradiation.

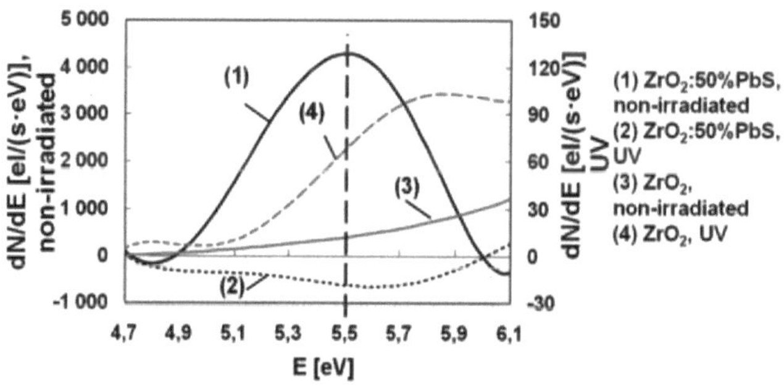

Fig. 2 Derivatives of the PE current of non-irradiated and 50 minutes with UV irradiated ZrO_2:50%PbS nanofilms and ZrO_2 matrix

In order to analyze the influence of concentration of PbS on the PE current, derivatives of ZrO_2:50%PbS and ZrO_2:20%PbS were compared (Fig. 3). Non-irradiated ZrO_2:20%PbS nanofilms have an inflection point at 5.5 eV which means that electron emission centers exist at this energy; however, concentration of the centers is less than in case of 50% PbS and is insufficient to provide well-defined emission maximum. After irradiation with UV, concentration of the emission centers in ZrO_2:20%PbS decreases, which is similar behavior as in the ZrO_2:50%PbS.

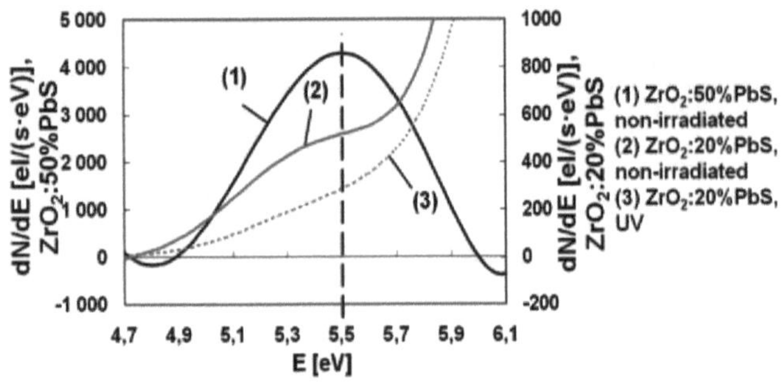

Fig. 3 Derivatives of the PE current of non-irradiated ZrO_2:50%PbS and ZrO_2:20%PbS nanofilms, and 50 minutes with UV irradiated ZrO_2:20%PbS nanofilms

It was found that increment of PE current $\delta N = N_{5.5eV} - N_{4.9eV}$ in the energy range from 4.9 eV to 5.5 eV decreases under influence of UV exposure for ZrO_2:50%PbS and ZrO_2:20%PbS nanofilms (Fig. 4). The energy range 4.9–5.5 eV corresponds to half-width of the maximum at 5.5 eV.

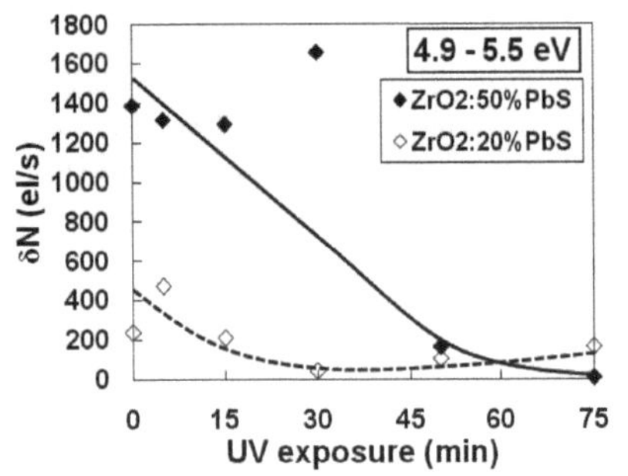

Fig. 4 Increment of PE current in energy range from 4.9 to 5.5 eV under influence of UV exposure

The dose-dependent changes of the increment of PE current δN were further analyzed in experiments with electron radiation.

B. Influence of electron radiation

PE from ZrO_2:20%PbS nanofilms was recorded before and after irradiation with electrons. It was found that intensity of PE current decreases after the irradiation (Fig. 5):

$$\Delta N = \frac{N_{Gy} - N_0}{N_{Gy}} \cdot 100\% \qquad (1)$$

where N_0 and N_{Gy} is PE current before and after the irradiation.

Change of increment δN in energy range from 4.9 to 5.5 eV after irradiation:

$$\Delta(\delta N) = \delta N_{Gy} - \delta N_0 \qquad (2)$$

where δN_0 and δN_{Gy} are the increments of PE spectra in energy range from 4.9 to 5.5 eV before and after the irradiation.

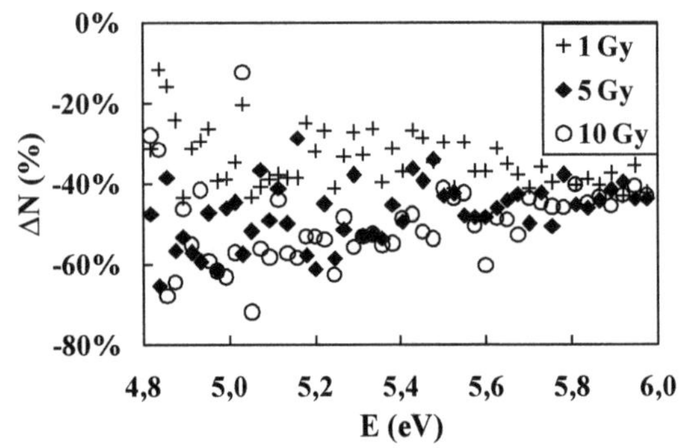

Fig. 5 Decrease of PE current after irradiation with different doses of electron radiation

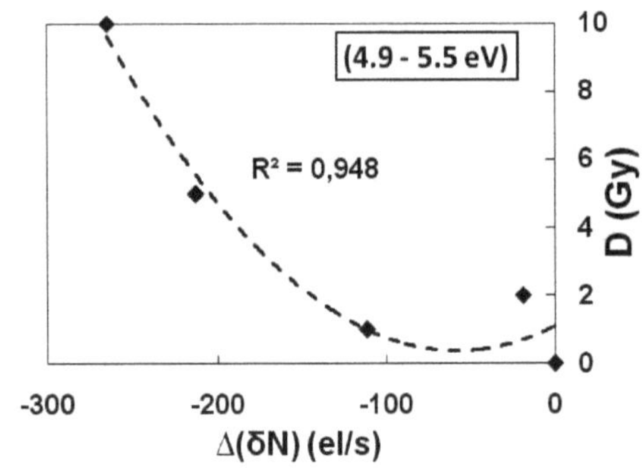

Fig. 6 Decrease of the area below PE spectra of ZrO_2:20%PbS nanofilms in energy range 4.9–5.5 eV after irradiation with different doses of electron radiation

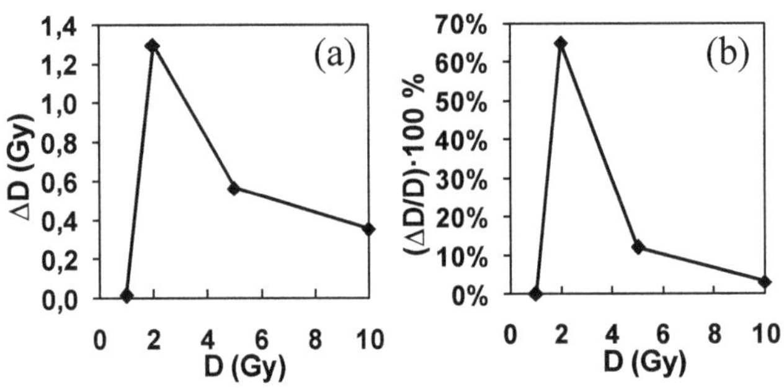

Fig. 7 Error of dose measurement depending on the dose of electron radiation delivered to ZrO_2:20%PbS nanofilms: (a) absolute values; (b) relative values

Second degree polynomial relationship was observed between Δ(δN) and the delivered dose of electron radiation (Fig. 6). In order to determine the error of dose measurement, theoretical dose $D_{theor\,i}$ was calculated for each delivered dose D_i using the polynomial equation describing the observed relationship. Constants of the polynomial equation were calculated using *Ms Excel* LINEST function:

$$D_{theor} = 0{,}0002168 \cdot \Delta(\delta N)^2 + 0{,}02517 \cdot \Delta(\delta N) + 1{,}1009 \quad (3)$$

Error of dose measurement ΔD_i for each delivered dose D_i:

$$\Delta D_i = \left| D_{theor\,i} - D_i \right| \quad (4)$$

Dependence of the error ΔD on the delivered dose of electron radiation is plotted in Fig. 7(a). ΔD decreases with increase in the delivered dose.

The relative error of dose measurement (Fig. 7 (b)):

$$\frac{\Delta D_i}{D_i} \cdot 100\% \quad (3)$$

Relative dose measurement error decreases from 65% to 11% when the delivered dose increases from 2 Gy to 5 Gy and doesn't exceed 11% in the dose range of 5–10 Gy.

V. CONCLUSIONS

Dose-dependent signal has been extracted from PE spectra of ZrO_2:PbS nanofilms. The signal is supplied by PbS nanoparticles and it is decrease of increment of PE current in energy range from 4.9 eV to 5.5 eV after radiation. Second degree polynomial relationship has been observed between the delivered dose of 9 MeV electron radiation and decrease of the increment. Error of dose measurement has been calculated for each delivered dose of electron radiation in dose range 0–10 Gy. It was found that error of dose measurement decreases with increase of the dose. Relative dose measurement error decreases from 65% to 11% when the delivered dose increases from 2 Gy to 5 Gy and doesn't exceed 11% in the dose range of 5–10 Gy. ZrO_2:PbS nanofilms have promising application in nanodosimetry of ionizing radiation. However, further adjustment of the method of dose reading is required in order to reduce dose measurement error to 1%.

ACKNOWLEDGMENT

This work has been supported by the European Social Fund within the project «Support for the implementation of doctoral studies at Riga Technical University – 2» No. 2011/0053/1DP/1.1.2.1.2/11/IPIA/VIAA/003.

CONFLICT OF INTEREST

The authors declare that they have no conflict of interest.

REFERENCES

1. Nettelbeck H, Rabus H (2011) Nanodosimetry: The missing link between radiobiology and radiation physics? Radiat Meas 46:893-897
2. Fuks E, Horowitz Y S, Horowitz A et al. (2011) Thermoluminescence solid-state nanodosimetry–the peak 5a/5 dosemeter. Radiat Prot Dosim 143:416-426
3. Ibach H (1977) Electron Spectroscopy for Surface Analysis. Springer Berlin Heidelberg
4. Dekhtyar Yu (2013) Emission of weak elections: Dosimetry of nanovolumes. Radiat Meas 55:34-37
5. Sashchiuk A, Lifshitz E, Reisfeld R et al (2002) Optical and conductivity properties of PbS nanocrystals in amorphous zirconia sol-gel films. J Sol-Gel Sci Techn 24:31-38
6. Saraidarov T, Reisfeld R, Sashchiuk A et al (2005) Nanocrystallites of lead sulfide in hybrid films prepared by sol–gel process. J Sol-Gel Sci Techn 34:137-145

Author: Marina Romanova
Institute: Institute of Biomedical Engineering and Nanotechnologies, Riga Technical University
Street: Ezermalas Street 6k
City: Riga
Country: Latvia
Email: marina.romanova@rtu.lv

Absorption and Scatter Properties of Tungsten Structured Composite Material

G. Boka[1], E. Reine[1], A. Svarca[1], M. Kuzminskis[1], S. Bikova[1], Y. Bauman[1,2], and Y. Dekhtyar[3]

[1] Riga East University Hospital, Clinic of Therapeutic Radiology and Medical Physics, Riga, Latvia
[2] Latvian Inventor's Association, Riga, Latvia
[3] Riga Technical University, Riga, Latvia, Riga, Latvia

Abstract- **Work was studied in the composite material (tungsten and ceresin composite material) absorption and scattering characteristics as well as comparison with until now used Bi-Sn-Pb compound. the hypothesis is that this type of composite material can be used as a substitute for metal alloy in radiation therapy. The aim is to determine the absorption and scatter of the composite, as well as to find out whether this kind of material can be applied to radiation therapy.**

Keywords – **Composite, Tungsten, Radiation shielding, electron beam**

I. Introduction

Today, radiation therapy as a treatment method occupies an increasingly important role. Consequently, it is also growing demand for higher precision treatment goal - capable of sufficiently large doses of radiation target volume and at the same time as little damaging healthy tissue structures. Electrons are the particles that are generally used in routine clinics [1]. In more complex cases for electron treatments, when it is necessary to protect the tumor intact organs, but they are located too close to the target, amount of exposure to healthy tissue is inevitable. In this cases additionally use metal masks that are made of alloy Bi-Pb-Sn material and has a high absorption, relatively low dispersion. But the manufacturing process of this shielding material is long and complex, as well as lead, of course, is a toxic material.

II. Purpose / objective

To measure and compare Bi-Pb-Sn alloy transmission factors with new tungsten-ceresin structured composite material for radiation therapy purposes for complicated tumor locations and surrounded tissues protection from radiation.

III. Materials and methods

A. Test preparation.

Work was studied in the composite material (tungsten and ceresin composite material) absorption and scattering characteristics as well as comparison with until now used Bi-Sn-Pb compound. The hypothesis is that this type of composite material can be used as a substitute for metal alloy in radiation therapy. The aim is to determine the absorption and scatter of the composite, as well as to find out whether this kind of material can be applied to radiation therapy. Thickness of specimen is 1 cm.

B. Measurement of absorbtion

Transmission factors measurements were made for electron radiation supplied from a linear accelerator Clinac 2100C/D (Varian Medical Systems, USA). The metallic and composite specimens were exposed with 4, 6, 9, 12, 16, 20MeV electron energies, dose rate 300 MU/min, and dose 2Gy to a depth of each energy dose maximum. In addition the composite was exposed with the dose rates 100, 300, 600MU/min.

An incident radiation beam was perpendicular to the surface of a solid water phantom, where the specimens were located . The Dose measurements were performed at the region of high doses – effective point of measurement (Table 1) and source-axis distance (SAD) 100cm. Radiation detector Scanditronix Wellhöfer plane parallel ion-chamber [2] type PPC05 with its active volume 0.05 cm^3 [3] was used. Measurements were performed five times for each energy, dose rate, and the specimen.

Table 1 Detector depth at the water equivalent phantom

Electron energy, MeV	Effective point of measurement, mm
4	5
6	11
9	19
12	26
16	26
20	24

Á. Jobbágy (ed.), *First European Biomedical Engineering Conference for Young Investigators*,
IFMBE Proceedings 50, DOI: 10.1007/978-981-287-573-0_15

C. *Measurement of scattering.*

The planar dose distributions perpendicular to the central axis and along axis dose were measured by using a Gafchromic EBT2 films in solid water phantom.

Fig. 1 Electron beam calibration film scanner output.

During measurements calibration films 5×25,4 cm^2 were placed at an SAD of 100 cm and at considering depth using plates (30 × 30 cm^2, set of different thicknesses) of Solid Water phantom. Film was irradiated with 4 × 4 cm^2 field. For calibration purposes, at least 6 films irradiated doses ranging between 0,5 and 3 Gy (Fig.1). The scans of the images of the exposed film were acquired with RGB Canon ScanLide100 scanner. The response of the scanner is matched to the absorbance of the dosimetry film [4]. For reconstruction of image information only red color channel was used. Considering that for doses up to 3 Gy, scanner provides the most sensitive response for EBT2 film from red colour channel. For all the sessions film orientation during the scan was in fixed condition. The scanner output resolution was set to 75 dpi. Software based image corrections and filters were not applied. Acquisition and analysis of images was performed using PTW (Freiburg, Germany) software. Doses distributions were calculated using an obtained Optical density - Dose calibration curves.

IV. Results

Composite and metal transmission factor is independent on the dose rate value changes (Fig.1). Figure 2 shows a set of metal alloy and composite transmission measurements using the 5 electron energies. Transmission coefficient for composite material is acceptable for electron energies 4MeV (0,34%), 6MeV (0,78%), 9MeV (1,5%) and 12MeV(2,66%), based on the fact that the shield should be chosen on the basis of allowable transmission (5%) [5] At 16MeV (5,7%) and 20MeV (18,21%) transmission coefficient significantly exceeds the value of 5%. At energies 4MeV(0,08%), 6MeV(0,15%), 9MeV(0,25%) and 12MeV (0,5%) transmission difference between metal and composite materials does not significant in contrast to the 16MeV (1,4%) and 20MeV (11%). Analyzing the adjoin scattering edges effects we got that in 2 mm depth the dose distribution on the surface near block edges for metal alloy is more than with composite block generated. Therefore the difference in dose between the metal and composite block material could be calculated as:

$$\frac{\text{Dose of metal block generated field} - \text{Dose of composite block generated field}}{\text{Dose of metal block generated field}}$$

,assuming that the metal alloy is the etalon (Fig.3, Fig.4). The maximum difference being 0,27 Gy (13,5% of prescription dose) and 0,13 Gy (6,5%) for the 4MeV and 16 Mev electron energies respectively.

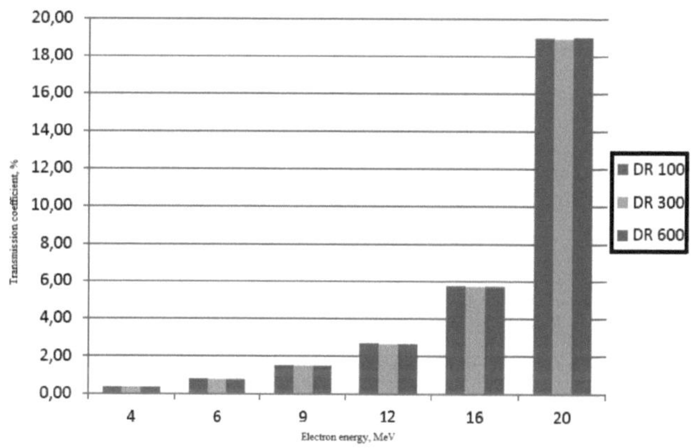

Fig.1 Metal alloy and composite material transmission factor comparison for different dose rate values.

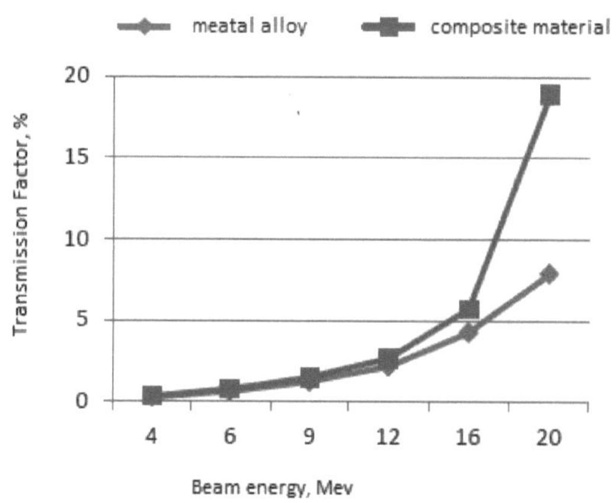

Fig. 2 Metal alloy and composite material transmission factors comparison for different electron beams.

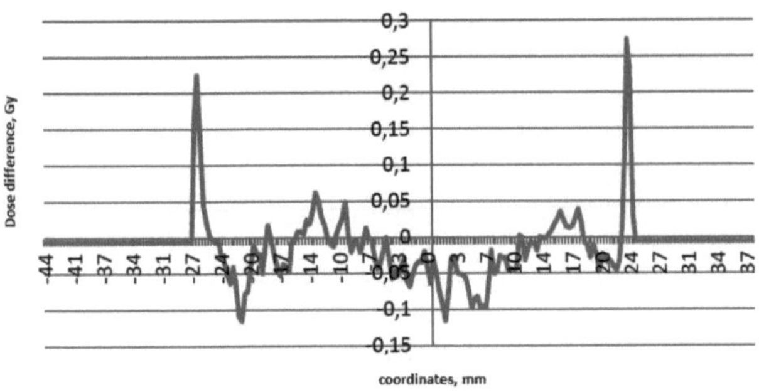

Fig. 3 Metal alloy and composite material Dose comparison for 4MeV electron beam

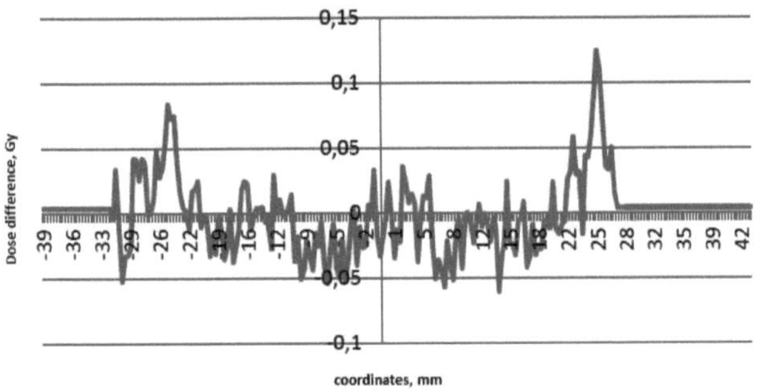

Fig. 4 Metal alloy and composite material Dose comparison for 16MeV electron beam

V. Conclusions

According to the attenuation of tungsten structured composite material can be effective and safe material for protection of the patient against radiation It can help to provide a high targeting precision and can be researched for different composite material components and proportion. Further analyses is needed for the composite structure evaluation. This possibility has to be evaluated by further studies of dose – tungsten particle size (microsize, nanosize) relationships. Nevertheless, the study results are very promising and clearly demonstrate superiority of this compound.

References

1. M.Beyzadeoglu, G.Ozyigit, C.Ebruli. Basic Radiation Oncology, Springer 2010, p11
2. F.M.Khan, The phisics of radiation therapy (second edition), Williams & Wilkins, 2003, p560
3. Technical Data, Plane-Parallel Ionization Chambers, CNMC Company Inc
4. GAFCHROMIC®EBT2 Dosimetry film. Available from: http://www.gafchromic.com/
5. F.M.Khan, The phisics of Radiation Therapy (Fourth Edition), Lippincott Williams & Wilkins, 2010, p292

Author: Galina Boka
Institute: Latvian Oncology center of Riga East University hospital
Street: 4, Hipokrata str.
City: Riga
Country: Latvia
Email: galina_boka@inbox.lv

Towards Optically Induced Semiconductor Gas Sensor: Sensing of Acetone

Yu Dekhtyar, M. Komars, M. Sneiders, and M. Selutina

Institute of Biological Engineering and Nanotechnology, Riga Technical University, Riga, Latvia

Abstract— **Breath analysis is in use since a long history as a part of medical diagnostics. Idea that some of the diseases are characterised by a specific odour was already known since the Hippocrates time. Modern breath analysis has significantly developed comparing to the discovery of the several hundred different VOCs in the common human breath [1] to more than a thousand different VOCs [2]. Regrettably, lack of specificity and selectivity of the semiconductor sensors lead to complications sensing to differ between those compounds for modern semiconductor. Accordingly, it may be a challenge to give right diagnosis to a patient.**

To improve such a drawback, a new approach of sensing was provided. Using n- doped semiconductor and the spotlight lamp as an optical irradiation source have shown a possibility to sense different concentrations of acetone vapour. Measured signal maximal increment relative to air in the presence of acetone is 17% (measurement uncertainty 0,72%). It is possible clearly distinguish between healthy and diabetic patients. Thus present way of stimulation may be used to increase level of acetone sensing.

Keywords—**gas sensing, gas adsorption, surface phenomena.**

I. Introduction

Human breath tests in medical diagnostics have a long history. Since Hippocrates times it is known that patients with definite disease, have a specific aroma of breath. For example, incurable diabetes is characterised with acetone fruit flavour, but sulphur aroma is connected with problems of the liver. Nowadays, in 1971 Pauling et al. has noticed a large amount of compounds in exhaled volume [1]. Currently it is known that VOC founded in human breath is produced in blood due to blood/breath mechanism in lungs is exhaled [3]. Most of those concentration are particle per billion (ppb) or particle per million (ppm) [2].

Breath analysis provides new opportunities in the clinical medicine. Breath analysis is especially attractive diagnostic approach, because it includes non-invasive measuring of patient physiological state [4]. VOC verification in a small concentration is a very complicated analytical problem. Nowadays, in order to divide and define appeared gases in result of exhalation, it is used gas chromatographic and mass-spectral methods [5].

Despite the knowledge since many years before that exhaled VOC are disease determination, hypothesis proof was a very slow process, mainly because it is very difficult to define small concentrations using small devices [3]. Therefore, dealing breath analyse, VOC and its concentration can be used as biomarkers [6-9].

Acetone is exhalation marker for type-1 diabetes [10]. Healthy humans usually have exhaled acetones concentration in range from 300 to 900 ppb [11], but patients with type-1 diabetes have the concentration higher than 1800 ppb. In recent years, resistive gas sensors, that are based on semiconducting metal oxide films, are used for several breaths markers analyse [12,13]. This small difference between concentration's definition of healthy and sick people demands very sensitive acetones detector. Organic compound concentrations in human breath in the air are minimal and their determination to be accurate analysis requirements are sufficiently high. Such an analysis should be selective, sensitive, relatively fast and accessible, so that it can also be possible to use it easily at home.

Currently dedicated semiconductor sensors stand out with a high sensitivity and a rapid detection [14]. This characteristic allows to monitor and provide an early warning of the possible risks. In order to increase both specificity and selectivity for the semiconductor sensors a new approach is required. It is possible to make better on the assumption of dependence of the excitation signal following the parabolic law [15]. The result may be achieved by the use of optical transitions of electrons in materials of sensor.

Therefore to examine a possibility to increase semiconductor sensors efficiency optical stimulation took a place.

II. Materials and Methods

The main aim of current research was to carry out signal increment measurement and semiconductor time response in the presence of ethyl acetate vapour, n-butanol vapour and reference air separately using optical stimulation. The measurements were done using n-doped semiconductor.

For those purposes the test setup (fig.1) was built. The spot light source was used to provide homogenous optical irradiation on semiconductor surface. A regulated power supply was used to provide constant DC. To exclude the influence of the external conditions, such as room light and room airflow, the setup was placed in the chamber.

To produce signal increment characteristic the measurements were made at the certain voltage values of the power

Á. Jobbágy (ed.), *First European Biomedical Engineering Conference for Young Investigators*,
IFMBE Proceedings 50, DOI: 10.1007/978-981-287-573-0_16

supply (fig.1.). Signal maximal value was measured using a multimeter (fig.1).

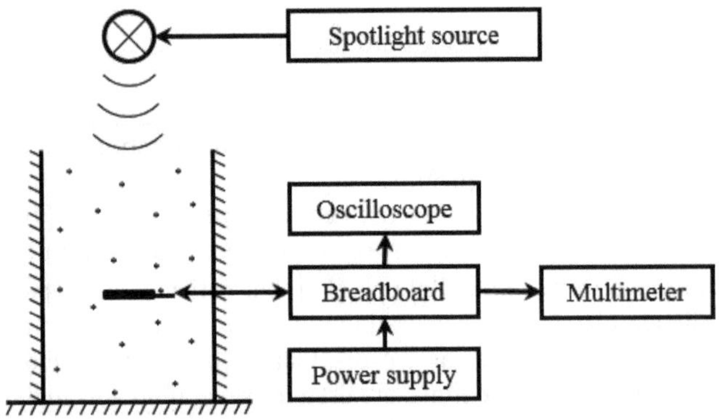

Fig.1. Principal scheme of the test setup. The spotlight source was used as an optical irradiation source. Source to surface distance was 210mm, the intensity 4500mW/cm^2.

Finally, signal increment (1) between vapours and reference air signal was calculated in the following way:

$$\Delta R = \left(\frac{Vpr-Air}{Air}\right) \cdot 100\% \quad (1)$$

where Vpr – the maximal measured value of the examined vapour, rel.val.; Air – the maximal measured value of the reference air signal, rel.val (fig.2.).

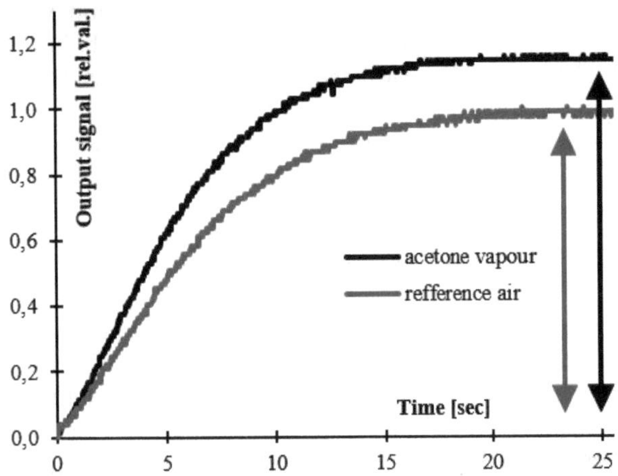

Fig.2. Increment calculation between vapours and reference air signal

III. Results and discussion

Measurement results are presented in the Figure 3. It shows a possibility for a stimulated semiconductor to distinguish concentrations of acetone in range between 0 ppm to 1,78 ppm.

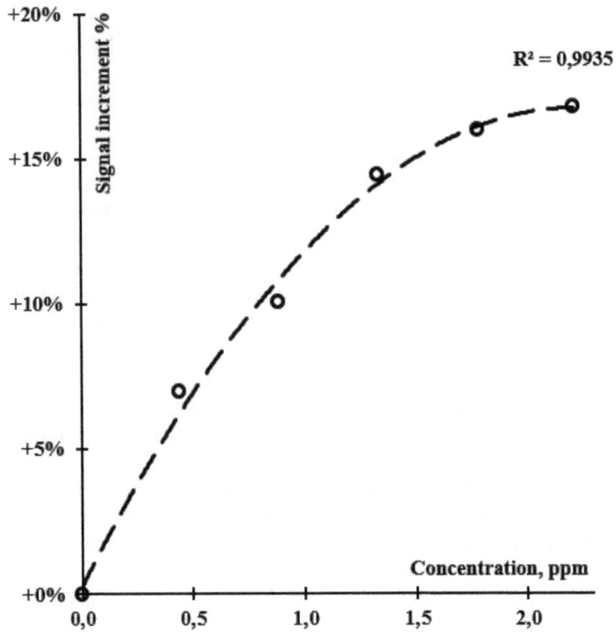

Fig.3. Sensor response for acetone detection (0 – 2,21 ppm)

Stimulated semiconductor response to acetone (fig.3.) is below 10% (<0.9 ppm) of signal increment for healthy humans and above 15% (>1.8 ppm) of signal increment for diabetics. This 1,5 times big increase in sensor response allow to fulfil diagnosis of diabetic patients by breath acetone monitoring with a portable stimulated semiconductor detector.

Acetone detection for healthy humans is linearly characterised, in turn to diabetic patient detection acetone sensor detection is slowing, which can be a source of sensor surface saturation.

Maximal measurement uncertainty value of signal increment is 0,72%. Maximal measurement uncertainty value of concentration is 1,2%.

IV. Conclusions

The defined difference in gained results shows that it is possible to use stimulated semiconductor to sense acetone vapour in range 0-2,21 ppm.

Patients with type-1 diabetes (>1,8 ppm) can be clearly distinguished from healthy humans (0,3 – 0,9 ppm), with calculated difference of 5,2% in sensor response (measurement uncertainty is 0,72%).

Sensor surface saturation was found at the concentration levels above 1,5ppm. Such drawback elimination will be studied.

Such way of the stimulation may be used together with modern semiconductor sensors to increase sensitivity. Nevertheless additional researches to determinate sensing threshold and ambient influence on the results are needed.

Conflict of Interest

The authors declare that they have no conflict of interest.

References

1. Pauling L, Robinson A, Teranishi R et al (1971) Quantitative Analysis of Urine Vapor and Breath by Gas-Liquid Partition Chromatography. Proc. Nat. Acad. Sci. USA, Vol.68, 10:2374-2376
2. Philips M, Herrera J, Krishnan S et al. (1999) Variation in volatile organic compounds in the breath of normal humans. J. Chromatogr. B 729:75-88
3. Marczin, N, Yacoub MH (2002) Disease markers in exhaled breath. Basic mechanisms and clinical applications. NATO Science Series, 448
4. http://www.omdiagnostics.com/
5. Phillips M (1992) Breath tests in medicine. Sci. Amer., vol. 267:74–83
6. Kim KH, Shamin Ara Jahan, Babir E (2012) A review of breath analysis for diagnosis of human health. Trends in Analytical Chemistry, 33:1-8
7. Chan HP, Lewis C, Thomas PS et al. (2009) Exhaled breath analysis: novel approach for early detection of lung cancer. Lung Cancer 63(2):164-172
8. Phillips M, et al. (2003) Volatile Markers of Breast Cancer in the Breath. The Breast Journal, 9(3):184–191
9. Shirau M, Touhaza K (2011) The scent of disease volatile organic compounds of the human body related to disease and disorder. Oxford J, The Journal of Biochemistry 3:257-266
10. Cao W, Duan Y (2006) Breath analysis: potential for clinical diagnosis and exposure assessment. Clin.Chem.52(5):800-811
11. Diskin AM, Spanel P, Smith D (2003) Time variation of ammonia, acetone, isoprene and ethanol in breath. Physiol Meas.24(1):107-126
12. Di Natale C, et al. (2003) Lung cancer identification by the analysis of breath by means of an array of non-selective gas sensors. Biosens Bioelectron.18(10):1209-1227
13. Wang L, et al. (2008) Ferroelectric WO3 Nanoparticles for Acetone Selective Detection. Chemistry of Materials. 20(15), 4794-4796
14. Elmi I, Zampolli S, Cozzani E et al (2008) Development of ultra-low-power consumption MOX sensors with ppb-level VOC detection capabilities for emerging applications. Sens. Actuat. B-Chem. 135:342–351
15. Dekhtyar Yu (2008) Photo-, Dual- and Exoelectron spec-troscopy to characterize nanostructures. Functionalized Nanoscale Materials, Devices and Systems:169-183

Author: MaksimsSneiders
Institute: Riga Technical University
Street: Ezermalas 6b, 248
City: Riga
Country: Latvia
Email: maksims.sn [at] gmail.com

Fall Risk Monitoring: From Laboratory to Portable Device, Influence of Sampling Frequency

P. Tamburini[1] and R. Stagni[2]

[1] Department of Electric, Electronic and Information Engineering "Guglielmo Marconi"–DEI University of Bologna Italy
[2] Health Sciences and Technologies–Interdepartmental Center for Industrial Research (HST–ICIR), University of Bologna, Italy
Department of Electric, Electronic and Information Engineering "Guglielmo Marconi"–DEI University of Bologna Italy

Abstract— **The understanding of locomotor stability is a critical issue in the assessment of subjects with high level of fall risk either pathological (e.g. stroke subjects) or elderly. Clinical assessment of fall risk is typically based on clinical rating scales; however, this approach heavily relies on the clinician's subjective judgment. Instrumental stability and variability indexes of gait can represent a promising solution for the objective quantification of locomotor function and fall risk. Furthermore clusters of stability and variability indexes give important information about the clinical deficits of subjects that could be the causes of the fall risk.**

An important step for the improvement of the assessment of fall risk is to analyze the subject's walk not only in the laboratory but also in his daily life. This is possible with the implementation of the stability and variability indexes in a portable device. Mobile phone is the ideal device for this goal. Indeed it is user friendly, cheap and although the IMUs mounted on standard smart phones have nothing to envy to other commercially available devices, but sampling frequency at 100 or 200 Hz is not compatible with the computational characteristics. The influence of reduced sampling frequency on the assessment of variability and stability indexes used for the monitoring must be assessed, and this is the aim of the present work.

The preliminary obtained results show that the influence of the sampling frequencies in the computation of the stability and variability indexes is not an obstacle to move the assessment and monitoring of fall risk from the laboratory to a portable device.

Keywords— **fall risk, fall risk assessment, fall risk monitoring, elderly, stability and variability indexes.**

I. Introduction

Falls represent a major community and public health problem, with large clinical and economic consequences.
The understanding of locomotor stability is a critical issue in clinical assessment procedures. Clinicians and physical therapists typically use clinical rating scales and questionnaires for fall risk assessment in specific population purposes. However, this approach highly relies on the clinician's subjective judgment [1]. More reliable and objective tools for the quantification of motor function and gait stability are needed. Instrumental measurements have been shown to represent a valid and objective complement to clinical rating scales in balance, gait and metabolic consumption assessment of both healthy and pathologic subjects [2-5].

Several variability and stability indexes were proposed in the literature for the subject specific assessment of fall risk. In particular, instrumental variability and stability measurements of stride time and trunk accelerations during gait recently resulted promising in the assessment of gait stability and fall risk in healthy elderly subjects [6]

Although promising, the assessment of fall risk without any indication of the subject specific factors leading to it, can not provide indication for the design of any effective clinical intervention for its effective reduction. Recent work [7,8] demonstrated that clustering appropriate selected indexes can provide indication regarding the specific subject alterations increasing fall risk.

The effective exploitation of this approach is meant in its implementation on a portable device for the continuous monitoring of subjects at risk, either pathological (e.g. stroke subjects) or elderly subjects. The ideal device to maximise the exploitation, and subject acceptance is a mobile phone. Although the IMUs mounted on standard smart phones have nothing to envy to other commercially available devices, but sampling frequency at 100 or 200 Hz is not compatible with the computational characteristics. The influence of reduced sampling frequency on the assessment of variability and stability indexes used for the monitoring must be assessed, and this is the aim of the present work.
This is an essential step for bringing the method from the laboratory to real practice without loosing the performance.

Á. Jobbágy (ed.), *First European Biomedical Engineering Conference for Young Investigators*,
IFMBE Proceedings 50, DOI: 10.1007/978-981-287-573-0_17

II. MATERIALS AND METHODS

A. Participants

Ten healthy young subjects, 7 males and 3 females (28 ±3 years, 174 ± 11 cm, 67 ± 13 kg), participated to the study. All the subjects were recruited from the students /volunteers at the University of Bologna.

B. Test procedure and measurement equipment

The subjects performed a walking along a straight line at self selected speed on 250 m long dead-end road wearing 2 tri-axial accelerometers (Opal, APDM, USA), one located at the level of the fifth lumbar vertebra and one on the right ankle.

Acceleration and angular velocity in vertical (V), medio-lateral (ML) and antero-posterior (AP) were acquired with sample frequency of 128 Hz.

C. Gait stability and variability indexes

Eleven gait variability and stability indexes were calculated on trunk acceleration signal during gait obtained from the walking trial. Such indexes were Standard Deviation (SD), Coefficient of Variation (CV), Nonstationary index (NI), Inconsistency of Variance (IV), Poincaré Plots (PSD1/PSD2), Maximum Floquet Multipliers (maxFM), short-term Lyapunov exponents (sLE), long-term Lyapunov exponents (lLE), Harmonic Ratio (HR) [8], which gives an indication of the smoothness of the acceleration pattern, Index of Harmonicity (IH) [9], Multiscale Entropy (MSE) [10], which is an indicator of complexity of the signal at several scales, and Recurrence Quantification Analysis (RQA) [11]. The two latter indexes produce 6 and 5 sub-measures respectively, based on the time scale in MSE or based on the feature of the recurrence plot that are analyzed in RQA, namely recurrence rate (rr), determinism (det), average length of diagonal lines (avg), maximum length of diagonal lines (max), divergence (div).

D. Data analysis

Stability and variability indexes were calculated on acceleration data from the whole duration of the walking trial.

Each indexes was calculated for the acquired signal (at 128 Hz) and for other two signals obtained from the original one by under-sampling at 64 and 32 Hz and also for anterior-posterior (AP), medio-lateral (ML) and vertical (V) acceleration directions.

Right heel strike instants were obtained from the angular velocity, around the antero-posterior axis, measured by the sensor on the ankle with wavelet analysis based method [13] and stride time was calculated accordingly.

The first and last three strides were removed in order to exclude gait initiation-termination phase.

The obtained indexes were testing with gaussianity test (Kolmogorov-Smirnov test) in such way was possible performed the right statistical analysis: ANOVA test with a p-value of 5%. Last step of the statistical analysis was the implementation of a multiple comparison analysis using a Tukey-Kramer test.

The statistical analysis compares the obtained indexes by original signal (the reference) with the indexes obtained by under-sampling from the original one.

Data analysis and statistical analysis were performed with MatLab (Math Works, NATICK, USA)

III. RESULTS

CV, PSD2, HR, IH, lLE, maxFM, rr and MSE for the time shifting 5 and 6 didn't show significantly differences varying the sampling frequency.

SD, sLE, det, avg, max, div and MSE for time shifting varying between 1 and 4 shown significantly differences varying the sampling frequency.

NI, IV and PSD1 shown significantly differences only for the sampling frequency at 32 Hz.

In Table 1 are reported the indexes that don't show significant differences (p_value>5%) and those that show significant differences (-), varying the sampling frequency at 64 and 32 Hz. The specific value of the p_value is not reported because this is not a result of a multiple compare analysis and also this is not relevant for the present study.

Table 1 Significant difference of stability and variability indexes at different sampling frequencies

Variability/Stability indexes obtained from signal sampled at 128Hz	Variability/Stability indexes obtained from signal under-sampled	
	64 Hz	32 Hz
SD	-	-
CV	p_value>5%	p_value>5%
NI	p_value>5%	-
IV	p_value>5%	-
PSD1	p_value>5%	-
PSD2	p_value>5%	p_value>5%
MSE AP $\tau = 1$	-	-
MSE AP $\tau = 2$	-	-
MSE AP $\tau = 3$	-	-
MSE AP $\tau = 4$	-	-

Variability/Stability indexes obtained from signal sampled at 128Hz	Variability/Stability indexes obtained from signal under-sampled	
	64 Hz	32 Hz
MSE AP $\tau = 5$	p_value>5%	p_value>5%
MSE AP $\tau = 6$	p_value>5%	p_value>5%
MSE ML $\tau = 1$	-	-
MSE ML $\tau = 2$	-	-
MSE ML $\tau = 3$	-	-
MSE ML $\tau = 4$	-	-
MSE ML $\tau = 5$	p_value>5%	p_value>5%
MSE ML $\tau = 6$	p_value>5%	p_value>5%
MSE V $\tau = 1$	-	-
MSE V $\tau = 2$	-	-
MSE V $\tau = 3$	-	-
MSE V $\tau = 4$	-	-
MSE V $\tau = 5$	p_value>5%	p_value>5%
MSE V $\tau = 6$	p_value>5%	p_value>5%
RQA AP (rr)	p_value>5%	p_value>5%
RQA AP (det)	-	-
RQA AP (avg)	-	-
RQA AP (max)	-	-
RQA AP (diverg)	-	-
RQA ML (rr)	p_value>5%	p_value>5%
RQA ML (det)	-	-
RQA ML (avg)	-	-
RQA ML (max)	-	-
RQA ML (diverg)	-	-
RQA V (rr)	p_value>5%	p_value>5%
RQA V (det)	-	-
RQA V (avg)	-	-
RQA V (max)	-	-
RQA V (diverg)	-	-
HR AP	p_value>5%	p_value>5%
HR ML	p_value>5%	p_value>5%
HR V	p_value>5%	p_value>5%
IH AP	p_value>5%	p_value>5%
IH ML	p_value>5%	p_value>5%
IH V	p_value>5%	p_value>5%
maxFM tot	p_value>5%	p_value>5%
maxFM AP	p_value>5%	p_value>5%
maxFM ML	p_value>5%	p_value>5%
maxFM V	p_value>5%	p_value>5%
sLE tot	-	-
sLE AP	-	-
sLE ML	-	-
sLE V	-	-
lLE tot	p_value>5%	p_value>5%
lLE AP	p_value>5%	p_value>5%
lLE ML	p_value>5%	p_value>5%
lLE V	p_value>5%	p_value>5%

IV. Discussion

The results show that the indexes calculated in the frequency domain (HR and IH) and those that describe the system as a whole (maxFM and lLE) were not affected by the reduction of sampling frequency, supporting the maintenance of the performance of the method when implemented on a portable device.

MSE can be affected by reduction of sampling frequency, depending on the amplitude of selected time shift: the higher the time shift the least the measure is sensitive to frequency changes.

V. Conclusions

In according to this preliminary study the reduction of sampling frequency splits the indexes in three different groups:

- Indexes affected by under-sampling (NI, IV, PSD1, SD, sLE and RQA)
- Indexes affected by under-sampling depending on the time shift use in their computation (MSE)
- Indexes not affected by under-sampling (CV, PSD2, HR, IH, lLE, maxFM and rr)

Indexes that belong to the two groups are those that, to the current knowledge of the authors, show the highest correlation with the clinical rating scales and provide indication of the subject specific factors leading to fall risk.

In conclusion is possible to affirm that the influence of the sampling frequencies in the computation of the stability and variability indexes is not an obstacle to move the assessment and monitoring of fall risk from the laboratory to a portable device.

Conflict of Interest

The authors declare that they have no conflict of interest.

References

1. Hamacher D, Singh N, Van Dieën JH et al. (2011) Kinematic measures for assessing gait stability in elderly individuals: a systematic review. J R Soc Interface 8(65), 1682-1698.
2. Sawacha Z, Carraro E, Contessa P et al. (2013) Relationship between clinical and instrumental balance assessments in chronic post-stroke hemiparesis subjects. J Neuroeng Rehabil 10:95.
3. O'Sullivan JD, Said CM, Dillon LC et al. (1998) Gait analysis in patients with Parkinson's disease and motor fluctuations: Influence of levodopa and comparison with other measures of motor function. Mov Disord 13(6):900-906.
4. Gillain S, Warzee E, Lekeu F et al. (2009) The value of instrumental gait analysis in elderly healthy, MCI or Alzheimer's disease subjects and a comparison with other clinical tests used in single and dual-task conditions. Ann Phys Rehabil Med 52(6):453-474.

5. Frazzitta G, Maestri R, Bertotti G et al. (2010) Rehabilitation in Parkinson's disease: assessing the outcome using objective metabolic measurements. Mov Disord 25(5):609-614.
6. Riva F, Toebes M, Pijnappels M et al. (2013) Estimating fall risk with inertial sensors using gait stability measures that do not require step detection. Gait Posture 38(2), 170-174.
7. Riva F, Tamburini P, et al., Motor stability evaluation in elderly subjects through instrumental stability measures and clinical rating scales. Conference proceeding pag .36 SIAMOC-ESMAC 2014
8. Riva F, Tamburini P, et al., Association between instrumental stability measures of gait and clinical rating scales in stroke patients. Conference proceeding pag. 146 SIAMOC-ESMAC 2014.
9. Menz HB, Lord SR, Fitzpatrick RC (2003) Acceleration patterns of the head and pelvis when walking on level and irregular surfaces. Gait Posture 18(1):35-46.
10. Lamoth CJC, Beek PJ, Meijer OG (2002) Pelvis–thorax coordination in the transverse plane during gait. Gait Posture 16(2):101-114.
11. Costa M, Peng C-K, Goldberger LA et al. (2003) Multiscale entropy analysis of human gait dynamics. Physica A 330(1-2):53-60.
12. Sylos-Labini F, Meli A, Ivanenko YP et al. (2012) Recurrence quantification analysis of gait in normal and hypovestibular subjects. Gait Posture 35(1):48-55.
13. Aminian K, Najafi B, Bula C, Leyvraz P-F et all (2001) Spatio-temporal parameters of gait measured by an ambulatory system using miniature gyroscopes. J. Biomech 35:689-699, 2002.

Author: Paola Tamburini
Institute: University of Bologna
Street: Via Venezia 52
City: Cesena
Country: Italy
Email: p.tamburini@unibo.it

Development of a Closed Loop FES System Based on NARX Radial Based Network

N.S. Popov, D.J. Đozić, M. Stanković, G.M. Krajoski, and D. Stanišić

Department for Systems, Signals and Control, Faculty of technical sciences, University of Novi Sad, Serbia

Abstract— **In this paper design of a closed loop FES system for torque control is presented. Snap power worker s used for measuring muscle torque. Using this system torque is proportional to angle of a flexion so by controlling angle of a flexion torque is controlled too. During functional electrical stimulation 3 parameters can be changed: pulse width, pulse amplitude and time between two impulses. In this paper pulse amplitude and frequency are constant and system is controlled by changing pulse width. PI regulator is used to minimize difference between desired trajectory and system output. Parameters of a PI controller are obtained by minimizing mean square error on simulated system. In this paper NARX Radial based neural network model of system is used for simulation. Result on a real system show that this type of control system can be used for torque control.**

Keywords— **Functional electrical stimulation, PI control, real time control, NARX Radial Based Network.**

I. Introduction

Functional electrical stimulation (FES) is used to restore motor functions of individuals after stroke or after spinal cord injury. During stimulation impulses from stimulator activate motor neurons which activate muscle motor units. Usually stimulator generates current controlled pulse modulated signals followed by an exponential compensatory pulse of the opposite polarity [1].

There are few basic types of control: open loop, closed loop and hybrid control [2]. Although FES is usually used without closed loop because sensors are unpractical, initial parameterization and parameter adjustment must be done manually by clinicians. If precise position or torque is required feedback loop must be used.

In this paper an able-bodied subject's wrist torque, produced by palmar flexion, was controlled with the FES controller to track a desired trajectory by stimulating Palmaris Longus and Capri Ulnaris muscles (Fig. 1). PI controller is used to precisely control torque produced by wrist plantar flexion.

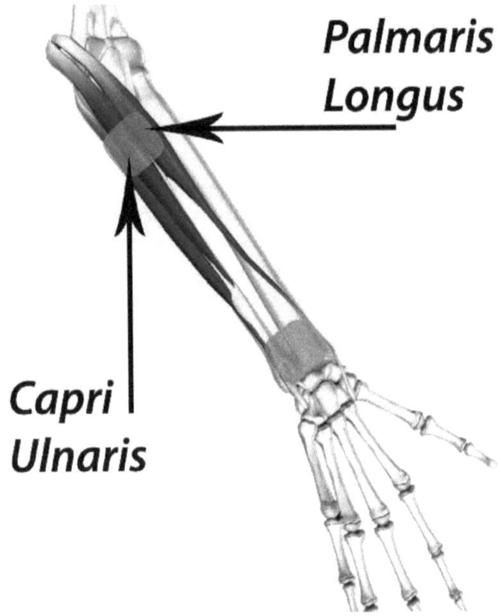

Fig. 1 Muscles stimulated by FES for wrist flexion and electrode placement

In order to have optimal torque control one must first have proper model. In literature there are many models used for FES from simple one [3] to complex one [4]. Complex models are more precise but identification of those models are more difficult and model optimization depends of proper initial parameters. In this paper we used neural network with radial basic function and NARX structure for torque prediction.

The experiment was carried out in the Biomedical Engineering Lab at the Department for Systems, Signals and Control, Faculty of Technical Sciences, University of Novi Sad, Serbia. The system performance of proposed algorithm was tested on three healthy, able bodied volunteer subjects (3 males, 27 ± 1 years old) who participated in the experiment after signing the consent form which was approved by the local ethical committee.

Á. Jobbágy (ed.), *First European Biomedical Engineering Conference for Young Investigators*,
IFMBE Proceedings 50, DOI: 10.1007/978-981-287-573-0_18

II. METHOD

A. System for torque measurement

System for torque measurement contains Snap Power Worker (SPW) and 3-Space Sensor (Fig. 2). SPW has four springs which produce counter force during wrist flexion. Torque of flexion is proportional to angle of flexion which is measured-using 3-Space Sensor.

3-Space Sensor estimates orientation of a sensor using Kalman filter based on information revised from accelerometer, gyroscope and compass [5]. It sends information about orientation to host PC every 1 ms.

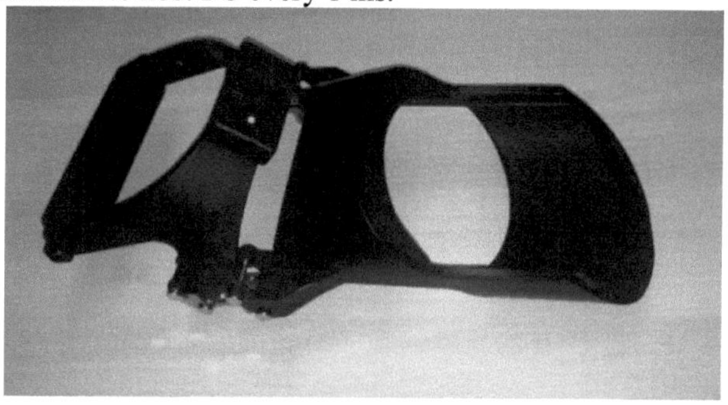

Fig. 2 System for torque measurement

B. TremUna

TremUna has 8 current controlled independent outputs that produce biphasic compensated stimulation pulses [6]. Each output has parameters presented in Table 1. The communication between TremUna stimulator and PC is realized via FT 232RL chip witch converts USB protocol into UART. FT232 chip is galvanically isolated from PC. Power supply is done by Li-Ion rechargeable battery which provides galvanic isolation of stimulator output.

Table 1 TremUna parameters

Name	Unit	Min value	Max Value	Step size
Amplitude	mA	1	50	1
Pulse Width	μs	50	1000	1
Frequency	pps	1	100	1
Delay	ms	0	10000	1
Number of impulses	No unit	0	10000	1

C. Experimental Setup

The experimental setup (Fig. 3) is comprised of following components: (1) Current controlled multichannel stimulator TremUna (UNA systems, SRB), (2) Snap Power Worker, (3) 3 Space sensor, (4) a standard desktop computer (host PC).

The control algorithm is developed using LabView, NI DAQmx and LabView real time toolbox. Data processing, modeling and optimization is done in Matlab. Communication with 3 Space Sensor is done in Microsoft .Net

D. System modeling

In order to have optimal control one must first develop proper model. In this paper we used NARX Radial Based Neural Network [7]. Using TremUna stimulator it is possible to control torque by changing frequency, amplitude and pulse width of an impulse. Torque is controlled by changing pulse width in range from 200 to 300 μs. Impulse frequency in all experiments was 50 pps, pulse amplitude is set manually at minimal value for which there is contraction at pulse width 200 μs. In order to obtain proper model for simulation, test input signal is applied and output signal is recorded (Fig. 4).Sample rate was 100Hz.

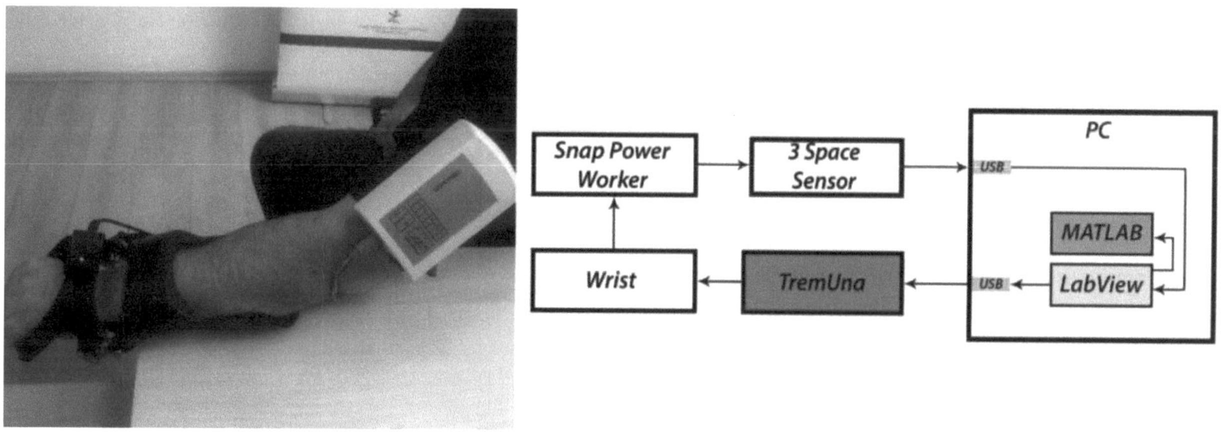

Fig. 3 Experimental system: picture of an experiment (left panel), block diagram (right panel)

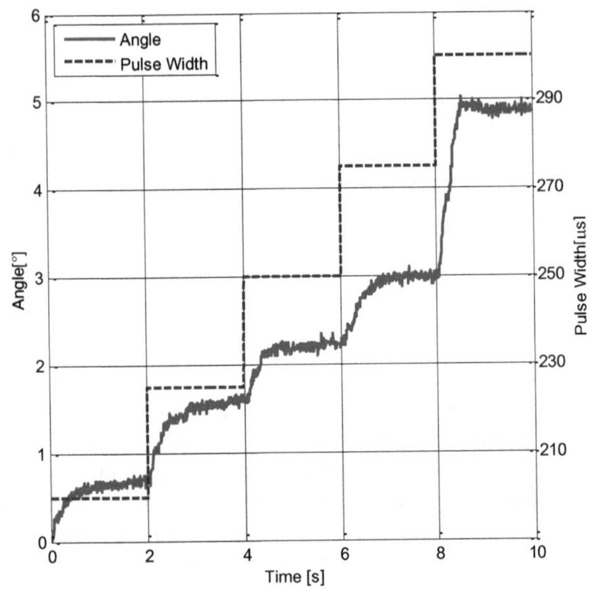

Fig. 4 Example of input-output relation for test signal

Muscle force output is usually modeled by second order system. In this experiment second order NARX model is used (Fig. 5).

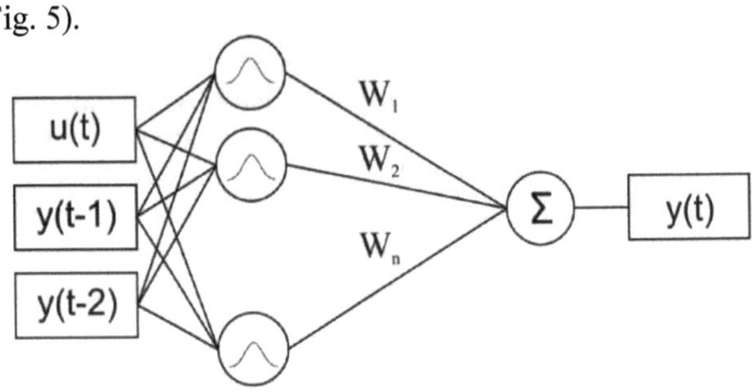

Fig. 5 NARX RBF Neural Network

80% of collected data was used for training and remaining 20% was used for validation. Least square error was used as the performance function and least square error was criterion for validation. Number of neurons in hidden layer is determined by training 10 networks with 1 to 10 neurons in hidden layer and later using one with smallest mean square error on whole set(training and validation). For all models, at the beginning of training, initial weights were set on random numbers. After that the training was done by Levenberg–Marquardt neural network training method. For every network training is done 100 times to reduce influence of initial parameters.

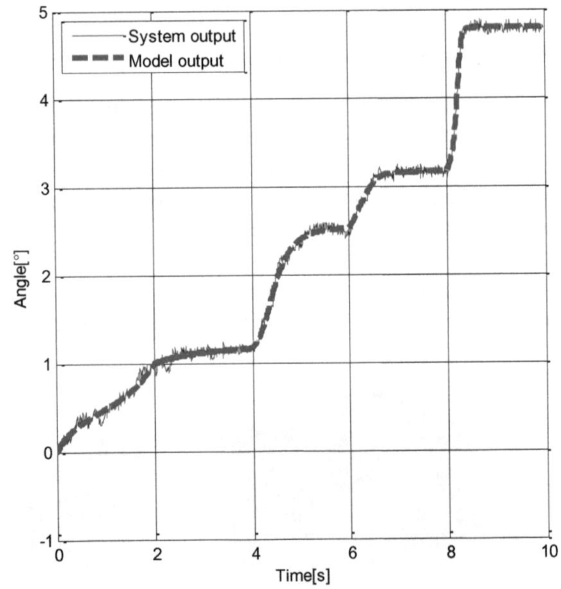

Fig. 6 Example of system identification

E. PI Controller design

Real time PI controller (Fig. 8) is implemented as incremental PI regulator with anti-windup, control loop at 10 Hz. It is used to minimize difference between set point and actual angle of flexion. System is simulated with constant set point and goal of optimization algorithm is to determent parameters of PI controller for which mean square error is minimal. Nelder-Mead simplex method is used as optimization algorithm. One may wonder why sample rate of control system and model is different (Fig. 8). This is because TremUna stimulator communicate with PC using USB communication and real time implementation isn't recommended at higher speed. Naturally model is more precise for higher sample rate.

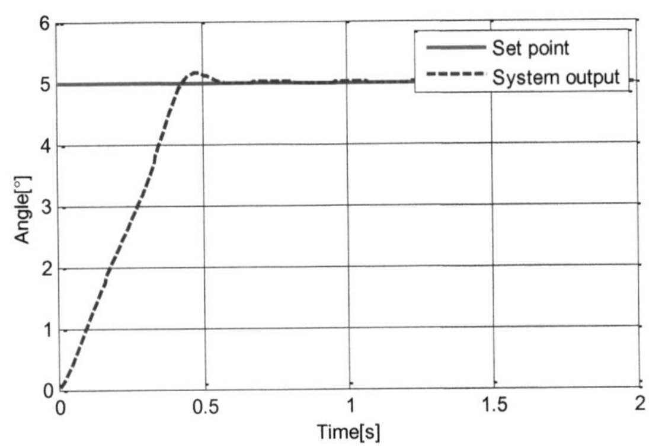

Fig. 7 Example of simulated system

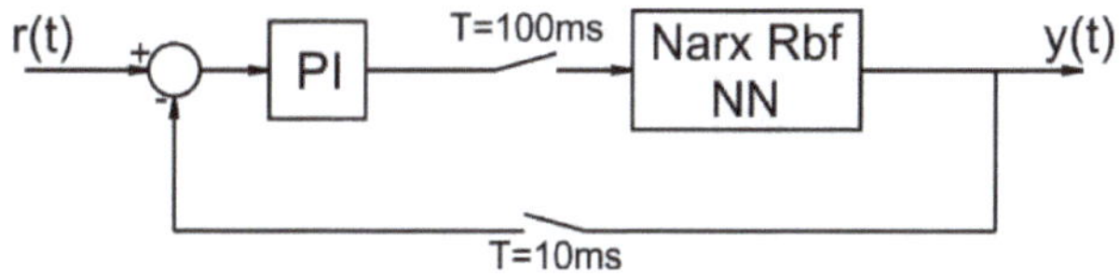

Fig. 8 Control loop

III. Resoults

In Fig. 9 is shown mean square error after neural network training for different number of neurons in hidden layer. It is obviously that for all subjects number of neurons in hidden layer is 3.

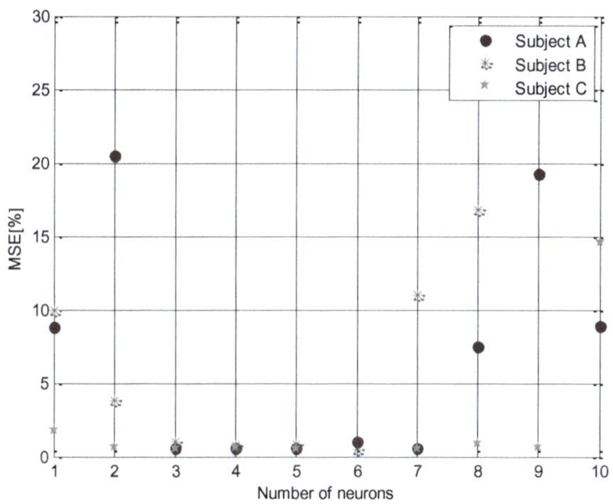

Fig. 9 Correlation of number of neurons in hidden layer and error after validation

In Fig. 10 are shown results after PI controller optimization and implementation on real system.

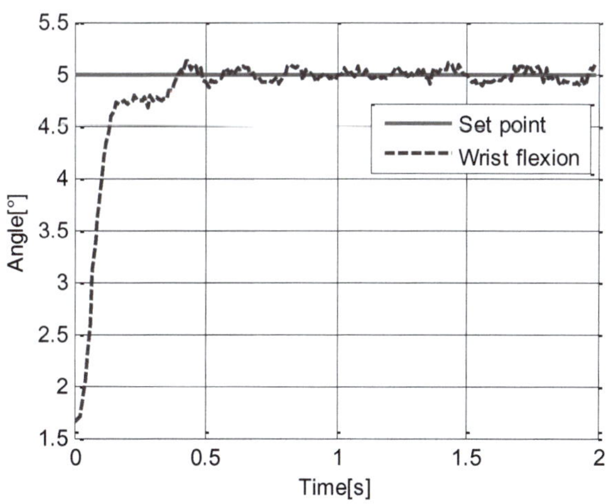

Fig. 10 Result of implemented PI controller on subject A

IV. Conclusions and Discussion

In this paper we presented algorithm for designing closed loop FES control for control of torque of a wrist during flexion. In our experiment torque of flexion is proportional to angle of flexion. Torque of flexion was controlled by changing pulse width during stimulation. In order to have optimal control NARX Radial based neural was developed. Model have one input (pulse width) and one output (angle of flexion). Parameters of PI controller are first determined-in a simulation based on a model and then implemented on real system for confirmation. Results on real system are similar as one on model.

Acknowledgment

This research was supported by the Ministry of Education and Science of the Republic of Serbia (Project no. III-41007) and by TEMPUS project 530510-TEMPUS-1-2012-1-RS-TEMPUS-JPCR “Assisting humans with special needs: curriculum for human tool interaction network (HUTON)”. The authors would like to thank prof. dr Nikola Jorgovanović for his expert advices.

Conflict of Interest

The authors declare that they have no conflict of interest.

References

1. Broderick B, Breen P and ÓLaighin G (2008) Electronic Stimulators for Surface Neural Prosthesis, Journal of automatic control, 18(2), 25-33, DOI:10.2298/JAC0802025B
2. Popović BD, Sinkjaer T (2003) Control of Movement for the Physically Disabled, Center for Sensory-Motor Interaction Aalborg University, Aalborg, Denmark, 2003
3. Bai EW, Cai Z, Dudley-Javorosk S, Shields R, (2008) Identification of a modified Wiener–Hammerstein system and its application in electrically stimulated paralyzed skeletal muscle modeling, Automatica, 45 (3), 736–743
4. Ding J, Wexler A S, & Binder-Macleod S A (2002) A mathematical model that predicts the force-frequency relationship of human skeletal muscle. Muscle and Nerve, 26, 477-485
5. Tong KY, Mak AFT and Ip WY(2003) Command control for functional electrical stimulation hand grasp systems using miniature accelerometers and gyroscopes, Med. Biol. Eng. Comput., 41, 710-717
6. Maneski LP, Jorgovanovic N, et al (2011) Electrical stimulation for the suppression of pathological tremor, Med. Biol. Engineering and Computing 1187-1193
7. Van Gorp J (2000). Nonlinear identification with neural networks and fuzzy logic, Faculteit toegepaste etenschappen.

Use macro [author address] to enter the address of the corresponding author:

Author: Nikola S. Popov
Institute: Faculty of Technical Science
Street: Trg Dositeja Obradovića 6
City: Novi Sad
Country: Serbia
Email: npopov@uns.ac.rs

Biomechanical Evaluation of the Stabilization Used in the Treatment of Distal Humerus Intra-articular Fractures

A. Kruszewski[1], P. Piekarczyk[2], K. Kwiatkowski[2], and S. Piszczatowski[1]

[1] Bialystok University of Technology, Faculty of Mechanical Engineering, Bialystok, Poland
[2] Military Institute of Medicine, Department of Traumatology and Orthopaedics, Warsaw, Poland

Abstract— **A stable fixation of particular bone fragments is crucial for the treatment of complex intra-articular fractures of the distal humerus.**

The presented analysis was focused on the evaluation of mechanical condition of a bone fracture union resulting from the usage of various configurations of the stabilizer. Numerical analyses (finite element method) were the main tool used in the research. A geometrical model of the fractured humerus (13-C1 according to AO/OTA) was prepared on the basis of CT-data. A simplified material model was applied to consider the bone tissue inhomogeneity. The geometry of the stabilizer was modeled on the basis of the VariAx® Elbow System (Stryker, Inc.). Two plating techniques: parallel (medial and lateral plates) and orthogonal (medial and postero-lateral plates) were taken into consideration. Loadings occurring during the flexion of the elbow joint were used during the analysis.

The evaluation of the global construct stiffness shows that there are no crucial differences between both stabilizer configurations. However, the analysis of relative displacement between articular bone fragments indicates that a higher stability can be ensured with the use of parallel plate arrangement.

Keywords— **biomechanics, distal humerus, fracture healing, modeling, plate stabilizer**

I. INTRODUCTION

The elbow joint requires a very early mobilization after injury to ensure good results of its rehabilitation. From another point of view, a proper stabilization of bone fragments is necessary during the bone fracture healing process. In this situation, an intra-articular fracture of bones forming the elbow joint should be fixed stable enough to ensure optimal conditions for the union as well as to make an early rehabilitation process possible. Consequently, complex intra-articular, multifragmental fractures of the distal part of humerus usually require a surgery to obtain a proper fixation. The gold standard in the treatment of such cases is the ORIF (open reduction internal fixation) with the use of locking compression plates (LCP) and screws[1].

Nowadays, two most popular plating techniques for distal humerus fractures are parallel plating (also named 180°), with plates located medially and laterally, and orthogonal plating (90°), with medially and postero-laterally located plates [2]. However, it is still unknown which configuration is optimal.

Fractures of the distal part of the humerus do not belong to frequently occurring accidents (0.5% of all adult fractures and 2% of all elbow injuries). Probably for this reason there is still no thoroughgoing biomechanical analysis of this problem. However, there is some research comparing orthogonal and parallel stabilizer configurations. Zalavras et al. used a bone taken from a human cadaver to perform mechanical tests of the bone-stabilizer system [3]. Penzkofer et al. used artificial bone models in their research [4]. Both abovementioned approaches allowed an experimental evaluation of the global stiffness of the bone-stabilizer system. However, it should be mentioned that reciprocal displacements between particular bone fragments are of crucial importance for the healing process. Such analyses were not performed in previous studies due to methodological difficulties.

The aim of this study was to elaborate a method for biomechanical analyzes of the humerus-stabilizer system which facilitate the evaluation of the displacement between particular bone fragments. The numerical simulation was chosen as the optimal tool for such task.

II. MATERIALS AND METHODS

The model represents one of the most common fractures of the distal humerus (13-C1 according to the AO/OTA classification). A reconstruction of the left arm of a 19-year-old female, made on the basis of CT-data, was shown in Fig.1.

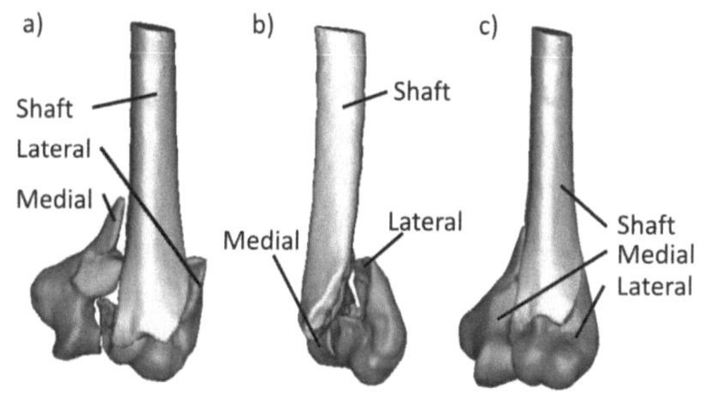

Fig. 1 Three-dimensional reconstruction of distal humerus fracture: a) front view, b) medial view, c) front view after reposition of bone blocks

Á. Jobbágy (ed.), *First European Biomedical Engineering Conference for Young Investigators*,
IFMBE Proceedings 50, DOI: 10.1007/978-981-287-573-0_19

Three main parts of the fractured humerus can be distinguished: the shaft – the biggest, proximally located part of the model and distally located medial and lateral fragments.

The model of the stabilizer was based on the VariAx® Elbow System (LCP) from Stryker. For the purpose of this study, screws connecting the plates and the bone were simplified and modeled without thread (screw modeled as a cylinder fully bonded to the bone in the thread region). First four screws used to fix the proximal end of both plates were modeled as a cylinder of ϕ2.75mm diameter whilst those placed in the distal region had a diameter of ϕ2mm. The location and the spatial arrangement of the screws were established in accordance to the AO rules and principles for the optimization of stability using screws and plates postulated by Shawn and O'Driscoll [5].

The model does not consider a direct contact between particular bone blocks. Such simplification ensures the possibility of evaluation of the bone fragment displacements only in regard to the stabilizer stiffness without consideration of the influence of reciprocal interaction between bone block.

Geometrical models of the bone–stabilizer system for both 90° and 180° configurations were presented in Fig.2.

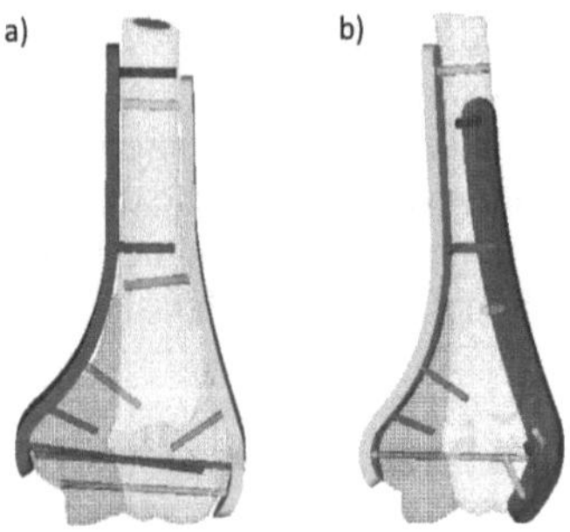

Fig. 2 Three-dimensional model of the bone–stabilizer system: a) parallel (180°) configuration, b) orthogonal (90°) configuration

The bone tissue was assumed to be an inhomogeneous, isotropic and elastic material. The variability of its mechanical characteristics was expressed by the use of different values of elastic modulus. Four sets of material properties were used to model: the cortical bone, the cancellous bone I (higher density), the cancellous bone II (lower density) and the marrow (Fig. 3). The shaft of the humerus was modeled of the cortical tissue and the marrow in the proximal region. The cancellous bone II was used in the distal part of the shaft instead of the marrow cavity (Fig 3b,c). Both medial and lateral bone blocks were modeled using the cancellous bone I tissue. The stabilizer (plates and screws) was modeled as made of titanium alloy. The values of material properties, taken from the literature, were presented in Table 1.

Table 1 Material properties

Type of material	Elastic modulus [GPa]	Poisson ratio
Cancellous bone I	1.5	0.3
Cancellous bone II	1	0.3
Cortical bone	15	0.3
Screws & plates	96	0.3
Marrow	0.001	0.3

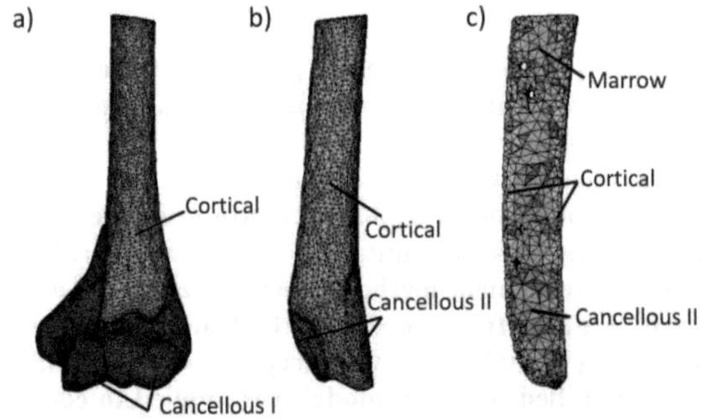

Fig. 3 Model of distal humerus after FEM discretization: a) all bone blocks - front view, b) shaft - posterior view, c) shaft cross-section (view from lateral side)

Kincaid et al. [6] analyzed the elbow joint forces associated with the activities of daily life. Based on their research, loading conditions for six positions of the ulnar bone versus humerus (elbow joint angle) during the flexion movement were calculated. The direction of the resulting JFR (Joint Force Reaction) used in the present analyses for particular elbow joint angles (0°, 30°, 60°, 90°. 120° and 145°) was shown in Fig 4. Loadings were applied on the trochlear surface. The value of the force used in the analyses was assumed to be equal to 200N, which well corresponded to the ADL (Activities of Daily Living) [6].

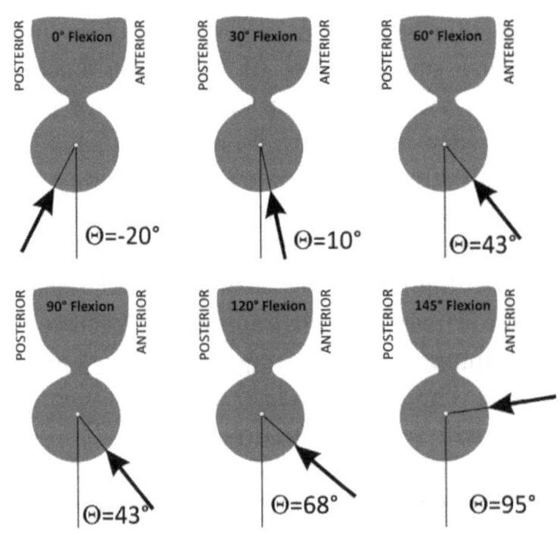

Fig. 4 Humero-ulnar JRF vector orientation (Θ) in relation to the distal humerus axis for six values of the elbow joint angle (based on Kincaid et al.). View in sagittal plane

It should be mentioned that directions of the JRF calculated on the basis of Kincaid et al. analyses for 60° and 90° elbow joint angles are very similar (43° and 43.3°). For this reason, the same loading vector direction (43°) was assumed for both abovementioned elbow joint angles.

III. Results

In order to provide the union of bone fragments it is crucial to stabilize them and avoid their excessive relative movement. The assessment of the global construct stiffness of the bone–stabilizer system was conducted using the value of the force acting on the model in relation to the maximal displacement occurring under loads. The results of such calculation were presented in Table 2.

Table 2 Global construct stiffness of bone-stabilizer system. Results presented for various elbow joint angles

Elbow angle	180°configuration [N/mm]	90°configuration [N/mm]
0°	150	170
30°	1626	1183
60°	156	145
120°	96	93
145°	79	78

A proper stabilization is especially important for the articular region, crucial for the future elbow joint movements. For this reason, the analysis of reciprocal displacement of the medial and lateral bone blocks was chosen as the optimal parameter for the assessment of mechanical conditions of the bone fracture healing process. A set consisting of 5 pairs of points was defined. Particular points forming each pair were located on the opposite sides of the fracture. Three of the pairs were laid anteriorly (Fig. 5a) whilst the other two were located posteriorly (Fig. 5b).

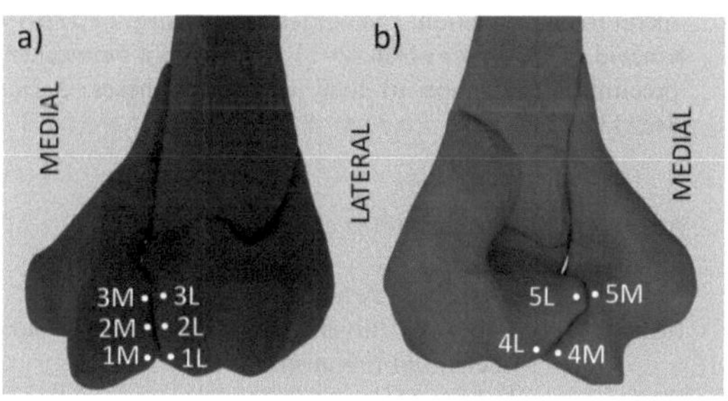

Fig. 5 Points used for the analysis of reciprocal displacements of bone blocks. Index: M - points located on the medial bone block, L - points located on the lateral bone blocks

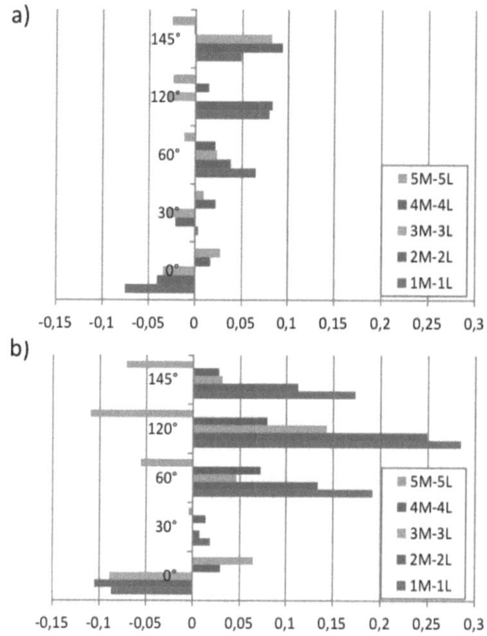

Fig. 6 Reciprocal displacement of the medial and lateral bone blocks in the normal direction to the surface of fracture for various elbow joint angles: a) parallel (180°) plate configuration, b) orthogonal (90°) plate configuration. Negative values mean an increase of the distance between bone blocks

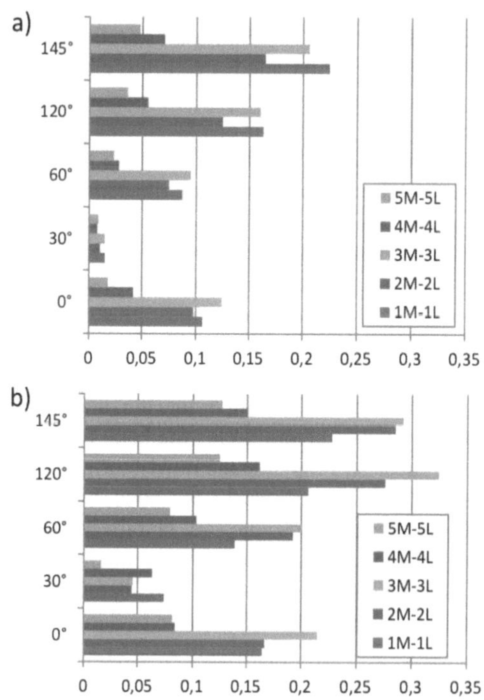

Fig. 7 Reciprocal displacement of the medial and lateral bone blocks in the tangential direction to the surface of fracture for various elbow joint angles: a) parallel (180°) plate configuration, b) orthogonal (90°) plate configuration

Reciprocal displacements between bone blocks were calculated for normal (Fig. 6) and tangential directions (Fig. 7) in relation to the surface of the fracture.

IV. Discussion

The evaluation of the global stiffness revealed that deformations of the bone-stabilizer system under applied loads were much lower for the elbow joint angle equal to 30° than for all other angles (much higher global construct stiffness). Such result was probably caused by the nearly axial direction of the JRF in relation to the humerus (the dominance of compressive deformation). The bending of the stabilizer occurring for the other JRF direction leads to a higher deformity of the system. It should be also noted that there is no significant influence of the stabilizer configuration (parallel or orthogonal) on the global construct stiffness for the analyzed loading condition. This observation should be obviously verified experimentally and such investigation will be conducted in the next stage of research. However, at present it is worth to noticed that discussed above effects and the value of the calculated stiffness very well correlate with the results of the study conducted by Penzkofer et al. They obtained 128 N/mm for orthogonal and 116 N/mm for parallel configuration under loading conditions similar to those used for the elbow joint angle equal to 120°, and 889 N/mm for orthogonal, 1126 N/mm for parallel configuration for the loading direction adequate to the elbow joint angle equal to 30°.

The analysis of reciprocal displacements of the articular bone fragments shows that all values are in the range below 0.35 mm. A higher mobility of bone blocks for the analyzed loading conditions may be observed in the case of orthogonal plate configurations. The values of displacement calculated for the normal direction in the case of orthogonal plate orientation were almost three times greater than for the parallel plate arrangement. It should be also noted that the values of tangential relative displacements of bone blocks are greater than those obtained for the normal direction. That effect can be unfavorable for the bone union because it results in a shear strain inside the newly formed bone tissue. Value and directions of particular bone blocks displacements probably depends on the stabilizer configuration (number of bone screws, spatial arrangement, etc.). However, this aspect was not taken into consideration in the present analysis, but is planned for future research.

V. Conclussion

Biomechanical conditions have a great influence on the bone healing process. This effect is especially important in case of the elbow joint where an early mobilization is necessary to assure a high range of movement after fractures.

The present analysis, similarly to earlier research, has not shown any important differences of the bone-stabilizer global construct stiffness obtained for parallel and orthogonal stabilizer configurations. However, our results show that even though the construct stiffness obtained for parallel and orthogonal bone plate configurations is comparable, the displacements of bone fragments relative to each other in the articulation are higher for the orthogonal than for the parallel plate system.

The results presented above have confirmed the need of a more detailed analysis of the multifragmental bone fracture stabilization and proven the usefulness of numerical simulation.

In the future, a further analysis is required to take into account more complex loading conditions (resulting from pronation/supination). There is a need of a broader analysis of various types of fractures. The future analysis should also include the optimization of the spatial screw configuration.

VI. Conflict of interest

The authors declare that they have no conflict of interest.

References

1. Goel D. P. et al. (2010) Open reduction and internal fixation of distal humerus fractures, Oper Tech Orthop; 20:24-33.
2. Sang-Jin Shin et al. (2010) A clinical comparison of two different double plating methods for intraarticular distal humeral fractures, J Shoulder Elbow Surg;19:2-9.
3. Zalavras C.G. et al. (2011) Biomechanical evaluation of parallel versus orthogonal plate fixation of intra-articular distal humerus fractures, J Shoulder Elbow Surg; 20:12-20.
4. Penzkofer R. et al. (2010) Anatomical plate configuration affects mechanical performance in distal humerus fracture, Clin Biomech; 25:972-978.
5. Shawn W. O'Driscoll, (2005) Optimizing stability in distal humeral fracture fixation, J Shoulder Elbow Surg: 14:186-194S.
6. Kincaid B. L., An Kai-Nan (2013) Elbow joint biomechanics for preclinical evaluation of total elbow prostheses, J Biomech; 46:2331-2341.

Address of the corresponding author:

Author: Kruszewski Artur
Institute: Bialystok University of Technology, Faculty of Mechanical Engineering
Street: Wiejska 45C
City: Bialystok
Country: Poland
Email: a.kruszewski@doktoranci.pb.edu.pl

Mathematical Description of Spinal Curvature Using the Results of In-vivo Measurement Systems

B. Jáger[1], T. Kristóf[2], and R.M. Kiss[2]

[1] Budapest University of Technology and Economics, Faculty of Civil Engineering, Department of Structural Engineering
[2] Budapest University of Technology and Economics, Faculty of Mechanical Engineering,
Department of Mechatronics, Optics and Me-chanical Engineering Informatics

Abstract— **The oldest and most accurate way of determining the shape of the spine is to make X-rays from two different angles, which can be performed once a year even in serious diseases, due to its high radiation exposure. However, in case of a conservative treatment of spinal disorders, continuous monitoring is necessary, thus different in-vivo methods are being developed, like optical (Moiré method), electromagnetic (SpinalTouch) and ultrasound based (Zebris) measuring devices, which can record the shape of spine without radiation exposure. The spinal curvature by the equation of a curve fitted on measured points of spine and by the complementary angles characterizing the spinal curvatures (thoracic and lumbar) derived from these aforementioned curves. Zebris and SpinalTouch measurements of 73 healthy patients –, aged between 10 and 15 – were the basis of the comparison. According to the results, the characterizing angles derived from the curves shows a high correlation (0.86-0.90) with the angles calculated with the traditional method, thus the application of these measurement methods and processing procedures can be reasonable.**

Keywords— **spine, spine shape, spline fitting**

I. INTRODUCTION

The regular examination of the posture of children is necessary to prevent structural and non-structural spinal diseases. The aim of these examinations is to diagnose these disorders as soon as possible to start the treatment early and then monitor the effect of treatments. [1-2] The easiest and most accurate way of determining the shape of the spine is to make X-ray from two different way, where the angles characterizing the spinal curvatures can be determined. [3] The Study Group on Scoliosis Orthopaedic and Rehabilitation Treatment (SOSORT) recommend to use X-ray once a year even in serious diseases. [4]

Due to the consensus and the risk factors, the way towards further development of alternative, non-invasive, radiation-free methods is opened. Nowadays many non-invasive spine examination methods are available (Moiré-method, flexicurve, inclinometer, kyphometer, goniometer, arcometer, 3SPACE, SpinalMouse, SpinalTouch, Zebris), which can be used for the measurement of the spinal curvature.

In our study, we examined data measured with the SpinalTouch (Department of Mechatroncis, Optics and Mechanical Engineering Informatics, BME) and Zebris (Zebris Medizintechnik GmbH, Isny, Germany) measurement systems, which are able to capture more hundreds of coordinates of the spine. Earlier studies calculated only the curvature of spine of few points [5-10], however the large number of measuring points gives a possibility for a fitting of curve. The goal of present study is to model of spine by spline curve fitting. We hypotheses, that this method provides more information on the spinal curvature.

II. MATERIALS AND METHODS

A. Theoretical basis of spline fitting

We used the well know technique the spline fitting for modeling the spine. During spline fitting a boundary value problem described in the following equation (Eq. 1) need to be solved where the *s* function minimizes the energy functional:

$$J[s] = \frac{1}{2} \int_a^b s''(x)^2 dx = \min \cdot \qquad (1)$$

The result of this minimization problem is a piecewise third-order polynomial function, which is C^2 continuous even at the control points. The advantage of this method is that oscillation does not occur, but a large equation system must be solved and every local change has a global effect.

B. Measurement tools

To perform the examinations on patients in standing posture SpinalTouch and Zebris spinal measurement systems were used. The SpinalTouch provides three-dimensional coordinates, beyond which the mobility, stability and load capacity of the spine can be determined in a special posture.

Á. Jobbágy (ed.), *First European Biomedical Engineering Conference for Young Investigators*,
IFMBE Proceedings 50, DOI: 10.1007/978-981-287-573-0_20

During the measurement the spine from C7 to S3 vertebra is examined. The device operates at a frequency of 150 Hz.

Zebris is an ultrasound based measurement device, which uses a measuring head with three ultrasound-based sensors and a pointer to determine the curvature of the spine. The distance between the sensors and the measuring head can be calculated by the multiplication of ultrasonic speed and the propagation time. The three-dimensional coordinates can be obtained by the triangulation method. This method provides 100 measurement points in each case, from which the values of thoracic kyphosis and lumbar lordosis are calculated based on the position of the processus spinousus.

C. Methodology of calculation

The curvature of the spine can be described with a function, fitted on the measured coordinates (coefficients, curvature, etc) and the angles calculated between the intersections of tangents to the fitted curve's inflection points. In sagittal projection the latter method is a better way to describe the spinal curvature, where thoracic kyphosis and lumbar lordosis are characterized by an angle.

Traditional method

The traditional method can be used to determine the characterizing angles of:

- *Thoracic kyphosis* by calculating the complementary angle between the lines passing through the first and second thoracic vertebra's, and the 11th and 12th thoracic vertebra's processus spinousus.
- *Lumbar lordosis* by calculating the complementary angle between the lines passing through the first and second lumbar vertebra's, and 4th and 5th lumbar vertebra's processus spinousus.

Regression line method

To determine the tangents to the inflexion points, a maximalization problem need to be solved, where the minimal and maximal slopes from the solutions of overdetermined system of equations should be determined, then the complementary angles between these regression lines can be calculated.

D. Examined patients

The subjects of our study were 73 children, aged between 10 and 15. The patients are healthy and/or treated with scoliosis. The measurement was performed on all the patients with SpinalTouch electromagnetic-based and with Zebris ultrasound-based measurement devices. The statistics of the patients can be seen in the Table 1.

Table 1 Statistics of the patients

	Average	Std. dev.	Min	Max
Age	11.926	1.203	10	15
Weight	48.978	11.929	26.5	91
Height	158.294	9.088	135	177
Total length of spine	438.751	35.500	356	534
Thoracic length	294.610	25.881	240	371
Lumbar length	106.373	13.896	68	166

E. Comparison methodology

Based on both measurement methods (SpinalTouch and Zebris) performed on the patients, we determined the characterizing angular values of thoracic kyphosis and lumbar lordosis, then we calculated the group mean, the standard deviation, the variance and the extreme values.

The angles calculated from our measurement data were compared with the traditional angles using the difference between angles, linear regression, the slope of the linear regression, the standard error of the regression and the Pearson's correlation coefficient as well.

III. RESULTS

A. Visualization of the results

As a result of the calculations, the outputs are displayed as shown by Fig. 1 where the blue continuous lines represent the fitted spline curves, the red dotted lines represent the approximate tangent lines computed using the regression line method and the traditional method discussed in Section II/C and the red circles represent the locations of the processus spinousus of vertebras, respectively.

It can be observed in the left figure that by using the regression line method the obtained three regression lines fit tangentially to the inflexion points of the fitted spline curve. The major advantage of the method is that reliable solutions were always provided even in case of small oscillations coming from the measurement process. On the other hand the traditional method often provides tangent lines not fitting tangentially to the spinal curvatures as shown by the right figure.

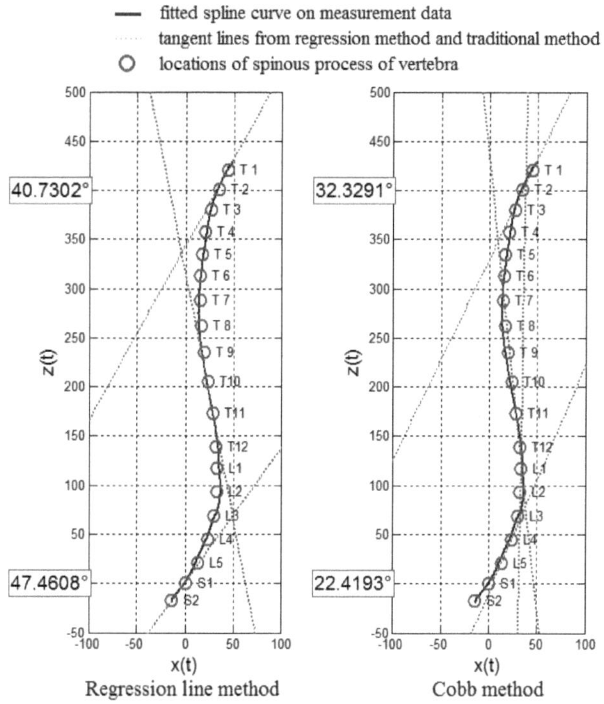

Fig. 1 Results of Zebris's data

B. Evaluation of results

The evaluation of the angles was calculated by methods discussed in Section II/C. In Fig. 2 the comparison of the results of the linear regression method and the traditional method can be seen. The red continuous line demonstrates the equality between the results of the methods. The red dots represent the angles characterizing the lumbar lordosis while the blue dots represent the angles characterizing the thoracic kyphosis of the spine.

The statistical evaluation regarding to Fig. 2 can be found in the Table 2.

Table 2 Statistics of the comparison of the calculation methods

	Difference of thoracic kyphosis	Difference of lumbar lordosis
Average	7.26°	20.10°
Std. deviation	4.56°	4.51°
CV	62.75	22.44
MIN	0.08°	9.57°
MAX	18.56°	32.90°
Pearson's correlation	0.86	0.90
Slope of reg. line	1.18	1.98
Std. error of reg.	5.46°	4.77°

One can see in Fig. 2 that the regression line method provides almost in every case greater characterizing angle values than the traditional method. Furthermore, comparing each characterizing angles the average difference between the angles regarding to the thoracic spine is smaller with 7.24° than in case of the lumbar spine where it is 20.10°. This observation can be also noticed in Fig. 1. High Pearson's correlation coefficients are received (0.86 – 0.90). The slope of the regression line regarding to the results of thoracic kyphosis is 1.18 with standard error equal to 5.46° while in case of the lumbar lordosis it is 1.98 with standard error equal to 4.77° (Table 2).

In Fig. 3 the comparison of the results of the measurement devices (Zebris and SpinalTouch) is presented using the regression line method. The blue and red dots represent the characterizing angles regarding to the thoracic and the lumbar spine, respectively. The red continuous line demonstrates also the equality while the dotted blue and red lines are the linear regression lines related to the two samples.

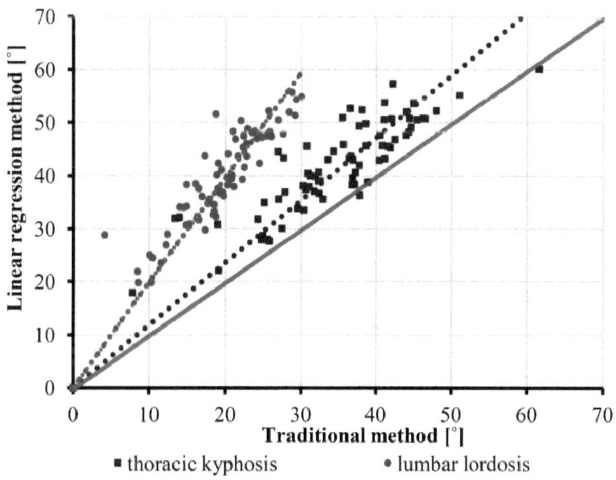

Fig. 2 Comparison of the calculation methods

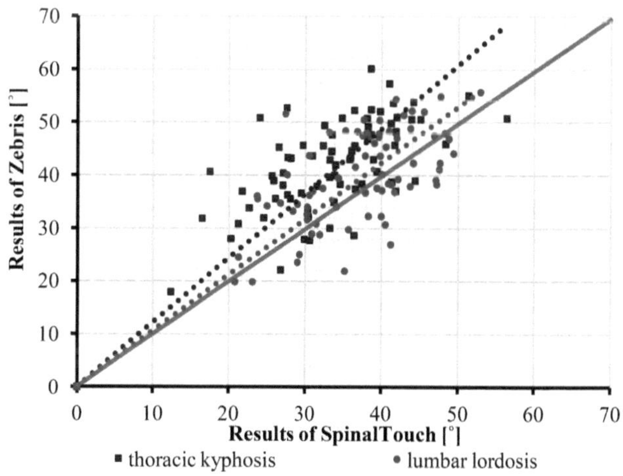

Fig. 3 Comparison of the measurement devices

The results show high deviation around the equality line which can be attributed to the perturbation of the same standing posture of children during the measurements and the layouts of the measurement devices differ from each other.

The statistics of data presented by Fig. 3 and summarized in Table 3.

Table 3 Statistics of the comparison of the measurement methods

	Difference of thoracic kyphosis	Difference of lumbar lordosis
Average	9.54°	6.46°
Std. deviation	5.80°	4.41°
CV	60.79	68.25
MIN	0.84°	0.02°
MAX	26.85°	24.26°
Pearson's correlation	0.61	0.60
Slope of reg.	1.22	1.06
Std. error of reg.	8.23°	7.50°

IV. CONCLUSIONS

In this paper a recently developed computer-aided method was introduced in comparison with the traditional method used in the praxis for the characterization of the spinal curvatures. It has been seen and understood that the traditional method does not consider the shape of the spine and the location of the inflection points which makes the measurement process easier. However, the developed regression line method provides results directly after the measurement process and the effect of the human error may be reduced. Furthermore the new method is based on the curvature of the spine therefore it gives more insight into the curvature of the patient's spine. The spinal curvatures calculated by regression line method provide greater values compared to values calculated by the traditional one. However, high correlations (0.86 – 0.90) were observed between them.

It is important to emphasize that during the rehabilitation process the same measurement method (Zebris or SpinalTouch) need to be used what was used in the screening test since the correlation between the methods is around 0.6 which can be also attributed to the difference between the layouts of the measurement devices.

Based on our measurement results, it can be concluded that the spline curve fitting and the characterizing complementary angles at the intersection of the tangential regression lines fitted to the inflection points of the spline curve can be a useful method for the screening of spinal diseases and for the examination of spinal rehabilitation process.

ACKNOWLEDGMENT

The authors wish to express their gratitude to Associate Professor Dr. Péter Tamás[2] for his accompanying useful advices and his helpfulness during the research activity and to medical doctor Dr. Mária Takács (MÁV Hospital Department of Orthopaedics) for the measurement data.

CONFLICT OF INTEREST

The authors declare that they have no conflict of interest.

REFERENCES

1. Zsidai A, Kocsis L. (2001) Ultrasound-based spinal column examination systems. Facta Universitatis. Physical Education and Sport 8:1-12.
2. Post RB, Leferink VJM. (2004) Spinal mobility: sagittal range of motion measured with the Spinal Mouse, a new non-invasive device. Archives Orthopeadic Trauma Surgery, 124:187-92.
3. Illés T. (2006) Gerincvizsgálatok (Examination of the spine). In: Szendrői M (ed). Ortopédia, Semmelweis Kiadó, Budapest, 218-223. (In Hungarian)
4. Knott P, Pappo E, Cameron M et al. (2014) SOSORT 2012 consensus paper: reducing x-ray exposure in pediatric patients with scoliosis. Scoliosis 9:4.
5. Malmström EM, Karlberg M, Melander A, Magnusson M. (2003) Zebris versus Myrin: A comparativ study between a three-dimensional ultrasound movement analysis and inclinometer/compass method. Spine 28:433-440.
6. Mannion AF, Knecht K, Balaban G, Dvorak J, Grob D. (2004) A new skin-surface device for measuring the curvature and global and segmental range of motion of the spine: reliability of measurements and comparison with data review from the literature, Eur Spine J. 13(2):122-36.
7. Geldhof E, Cardon G, Bourdeaudhuij ID, Danneels L, Coorevits P, Vanderstraeten G, Clarcq DD. (2007) Effects of back posture education on elementary schoolchildren's back function, Eur Spine J. 16:829-839.
8. Kiss RM. (2012) [Biomechanical modelling]. BME Faculty of Civil Engineering. TERC Kiadó 225-242.
9. Takács M, Rudner E, Nagy I, Jurák M, Kiss RM, Kocsis L. (2013) The new processing of the results of examinations made with Zebris WIN-SPINE spine-measuring method and its validation. Biomechanica Hungarica 4(1):29-37.
10. Kiss RM. (2008) Verification of determining the curvatures and range of motion of the spine by electromechanical-based skin-surface device. Periodica Polytechnica 51(1):3-13.

Author: Rita M. Kiss
Institute: Budapest University of Technology and Economics
Street: H-1111 Műegyetem rkp. 3
City: Budapest
Country: Hungary
Email: rita.kiss@mogi.bme.hu

Insertion Torque Function Analysis of Novel Dental Implant Geometry

D. Pammer[1] and E. Bognár[1,2]

[1] Budapest University of Technology and Economics, Faculty of Mechanical Engineering, Department of Materials Science and Engineering, Bertalan Lajos utca 7., H-1111 Budapest, Hungary
[2] MTA–BME Research Group for Composite Science and Technology, Muegyetem rkp. 3., H-1111 Budapest, Hungary

Abstract— **Since the discovery of the osseointegration implant stability has an increasing relevance. Determination of stability is particularly important for dental implants. Two types of stabilities give us information about the success of implantation; primary and secondary stability. There are many stability indicators, but their meanings are not exactly defined theoretically. The aim of our study was to examine and evaluate the insertion and removal torque of novel implant geometry in polyurethane artificial bone blocks with different densities, corresponding to the standard living bone density classification (D1-D4). Protocols given to implantation were followed during the drilling and insertion.**

With the analysis of the torque functions we found differences among the polyurethane artificial bone blocks. Torque functions showed us how the function's slope has changed the characteristic max-min values in different polyurethane artificial bone blocks. The drilling parameters highly influenced the characteristic of the torque functions.

Keywords— **Dental implant, primary stability, insertion torque, novel geometry, artificial bone.**

I. Introduction

Measuring the success of the dental implants is an increasing important factor; however there are many key details still unknown in the process of bone regeneration. Since the osseointegration (bone-implant contact) was discovered, one of the most important research topics is to determine and monitor the quality of the implant and bone contact [1].

The measuring of implant-bone integration is called implant stability measurement.

There are two types of stabilities; primary stability and secondary stability. Primary stability is measured immediately after insertion. This indicator estimates the initial success of the implantation. The following main parameters influence the primary stability quality: bone quality - structure and mechanical properties, the implant geometry and the parameters of the drilled cavity. Secondary stability is the result of the bone tissue regeneration and the quality of the contact between dental implant surface and new bones (osseointegration). Secondary stability measurements start after weeks of the implant insertion. The following main parameters influence the secondary stability: dental implant base material, type of the surface modification, bone regeneration ability, the state of health of the individual [2, 3].

There are many stability indicators as so many measuring systems to determine it. The nowadays used stability measurement systems have four groups.

The 1st one contains the systems which can measure stability in a non-invasive way. The 2nd one is the group of the invasive measurement systems. The 3rd and the 4th groups show which systems can determine primary and secondary stabilities [4, 5]. There are also standards for the implant stability measurement. The ASTM F 543 standard contains mostly the biomechanical tests of the bone implants (pull-out test, push-in test, driving torque, etc.) [6]. Some type of stability measurements (destructive measurements methods) cannot be used in living bone tissue, due to this there are polyurethane artificial bone blocks.

These blocks are solid foams (ASTM F 1839) [7], with different densities corresponding to the standard living bone densities (D1-D4) [8, 9]. The analysis of a new stability measuring system can be executed in polyurethane artificial bone blocks, cadaver bones and in living or not living animal bones. It is easier to work with artificial bone blocks, because ethical permission is not necessary for them. Artificial bone blocks can be used for the development of a new stability measuring systems as well. The polyurethane artificial bone blocks allow us to compare primary stability of different implant types in vitro and find the ideal geometry with the highest primary stability parameter.

II. Materials and Methods

A. The aim of the study

In this study the insertion torque and removal torque measurements are chosen from the different stability measuring methods. The measuring of the insertion torque during the insertion is obvious, because the dental implant must be inserted in the bone. The torque parameters contain a lot of information about the implant, bone properties and about the implantation procedure also.

The aim of this study was to determine insertion and removal torque functions of novel implant geometry in polyurethane artificial bone blocks with different densities.

Á. Jobbágy (ed.), *First European Biomedical Engineering Conference for Young Investigators*,
IFMBE Proceedings 50, DOI: 10.1007/978-981-287-573-0_21

B. Materials and instruments

Polyurethane artificial bone blocks available on the market were used for this research work instead of bone tissue. The use of these bone blocks in vitro is scientifically accepted [10]. Bone blocks with four different densities D1; D2; D3 and D4 were used. Table 1 contains the main properties of these blocks [11].

Table 1 Artificial bone block types

Artificial bone classes	Density (kg/m^3)	Analogue living bone densities (HU)
D1	~800	>1250
D2	~640	850-1250
D3	~480	350-850
D4	~320	150-350

To prepare the bone cavities for the implants the suitable surgical drilling kit and the drilling protocol were used.

Three pieces of Emotion Implant® were used without any surface modification. The novel implant geometry of Emotion Implant® has three main parts (Fig. 1) [12]. The root part has an aggressive large thread just as many implant types on the market. After this, the implant has the novel part, with cylindrical geometry and radial drilled holes. The aim of this part is to increase the surface of the implant with the design itself. The other aim of this part is to collect the bone grist, and facilitate the implant's bone integration. The main sizes of the implant are 12.5 mm×4.1 mm. The head part of the implant geometry has a small thread as many implant geometries on the market.

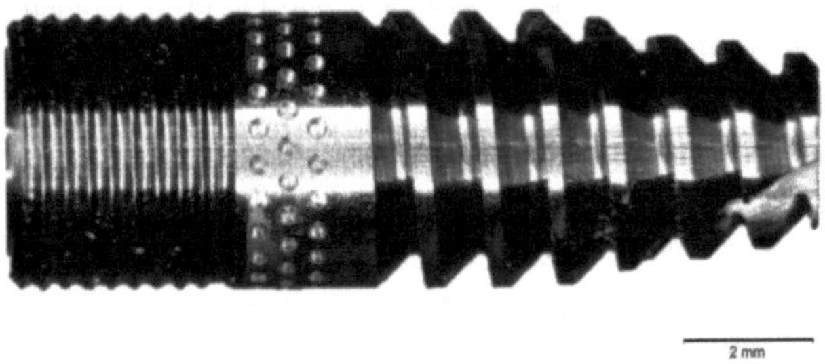

Fig. 1 Emotion Implant®

To record the insertion and removal torque values as a function of the rotation angle of the implants an Instron® 5960 tensile test machine (Instron, Norwood, MA, USA) with PTS torque measuring system was used.

For the microscopic analysis an Olympus® SZX16 (Olympus, Tokyo, Japan) stereomicroscope was used.

C. Methods

According to the drilling protocol three holes were drilled in each type of artificial bone. Due to this, different hole parameters were observed. The holes in block D1 had the largest diameter, almost the same size as the outside diameter of the implant. Holes in block D4 had much smaller diameter than the outside diameter of the implant, approximately similar to the core diameter of the implant. The holes in blocks D2 and D3 were among the others. By changing the hole sizes, we tried to ensure the best primary stability during the insertion.

The implants were inserted one after the other into the prepared holes (Fig. 2). The insertion speed was 25 RPM, which value is equivalent to the one in clinical use (Nobel Osseocare®) [13]. During the insertion of the implants the torque was recorded as a function of rotation by the Instron 5960® – PTS system. The same procedure was used for the removal torque measurements as well.

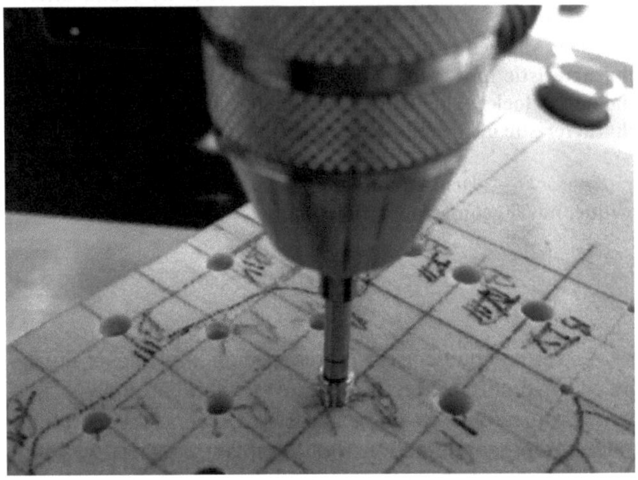

Fig. 2 Insertion of an implant in artificial bone block

Stereomicroscopic images were taken form the screwed out implants, and the cylindrical geometry with radial holes part was analysed. Besides, cross sections were made from implants for the two extreme densities, D1 and D4. The cross section was analysed with the stereomicroscope.

III. RESULTS

The microscopic analysis of the unscrewed implant's cylindrical geometry with radial holes shows that the holes are fully filled with polyurethane artificial bone grist (Fig. 3). This phenomenon arose with each implant independent of the polyurethane block's densities. This result supported the hypothesis and the expectation due to this novel geometry.

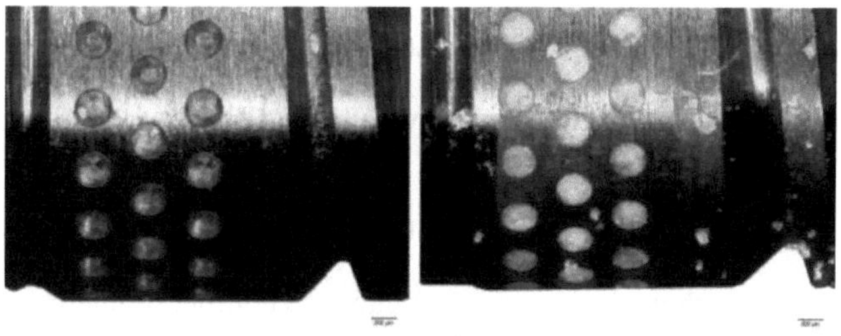

Fig. 3 On the left the empty holes on the implant surface and on the right the holes filled with polyurethane bone grist

The recorded insertion and removal torque functions of the implants were plotted (Fig. 4; Fig. 5; Fig. 6 and Fig. 7) for each block density (D1-D4). With the rotation angle values it was possible to calculate (knowning the implant geometrical parameters) the implant position in the artificial bone blocks. Due to this, the function shows the position associated with the current torque value.

According to the torque functions the results can be divided into two groups. The results of blocks with D1, D2 and the results with D3, D4 densities.

The functions of D1 and D2 show that the insertion torques highly depend on the diameter of the drilled holes. Due to this the minimal size changes in the hole diameters effected totally different torque functions. In the high density polyurethane bone blocks (D3 and D4) the results were influenced by the friction. Due to the large hole diameter the implants were minimally guided by the treads, and minimal deformation was observed in the polyurethane blocks (Fig. 8). The holes with large diameter showed that during the unscrewing the implants did not come out fully from the hole, but further turned in. The removal torque function shows this effect in D1 and D2, where it has a limit, beyond which the function doesn't decrease due to the torque of the friction.

The functions of D3 and D4 show consistently increasing torques as a function of the rotation. The nearly smooth functions show that the polyurethane artificial bone blocks have a homogeneous structure.

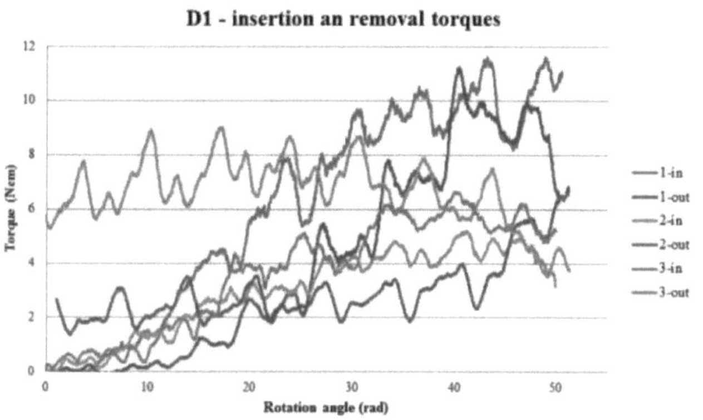

Fig. 4 Implant insertion and removal torque functions in D1 artificial bone

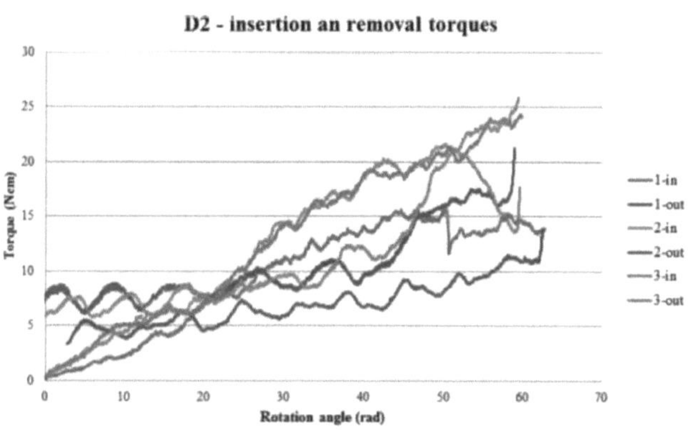

Fig. 5 Implant insertion and removal torque functions in D2 artificial bone

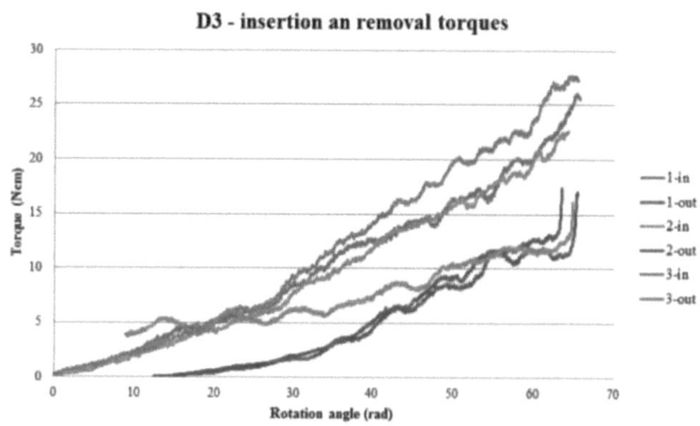

Fig. 6 Implant insertion and removal torque functions in D3 artificial bone

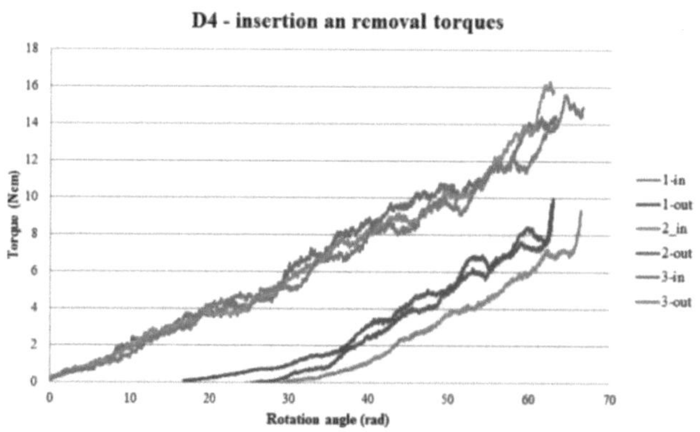

Fig. 7 Implant insertion and removal torque functions in D4 artificial bone

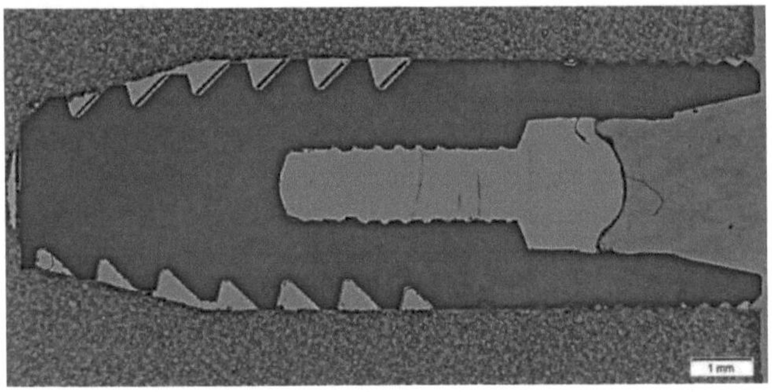

Fig. 8 Implant cross section in D1 artificial bone

Due to the small diameter of the drilled hole the thread guide during the insertion of the implant and the polyurethane artificial bone block had a large deformation near the implant (Fig, 9). Therefore, during the unscrewing the removal torque functions show a continual decrease until the functions reach the 0 Ncm torque value. The microscopic analysis of the cross section allows determining the deformed region near the implant of the polyurethane artificial bone blocks. The two extreme densities D1 and D4 cross section exposures show the different structural changes during the insertion. The deformation of the D2 and D3 blocks are in between the D1 and D4 deformations.

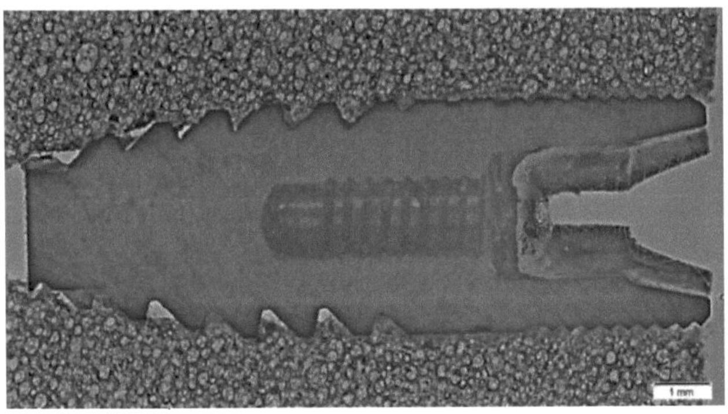

Fig. 9 Implant cross section in D4 artificial bone

IV. Conclusion

The functions of the insertion and removal torques gave us information about the geometrical parameters of the implant and about the artificial bone material parameters. Moreover the insertion torques give information about the inserted implant primary stability. The implant stability and the torque function characteristic are highly influenced by the drilled holes' parameter (diameter) in D1 and D2 polyurethane artificial bone blocks. The stability and the function characteristic are not sensitive to the small differences of the drill diameter in D3 and D4. Due to this the use of this novel implant geometry is recommended to D3 and D4 living bone types.

Acknowledgment

The used implants were provided by Radix Kft.

Conflict of Interest

The authors declare that they have no conflict of interest.

References

1. Adell R, Lekholm U, Rockler B, Brånemark PI (1981) A 15-year study of osseointegrated implants in the treatment of the edentulous jaw. Int J Oral Surg. 10(6):387-416
2. Elias CN, Rocha FA, Nascimento AL, Coelho PG (2012) Influence of implant shape, surface morphology, surgical technique and bone quality on the primary stability of dental implants. J Mech Behav Biomed Mater, 16:169-80
3. Chang, P. C., Lang, N. P. & Giannobile, W. V (2010) Evaluation of functional dynamics during osseointegration and regeneration associated with oral implants. Clinical oral implants research 21: 1-12.
4. Mistry G, Shetty O, Shetty S, Singh RD (2014) Measuring implant stability: A review of different methods. J Dent Implant 4:165-9
5. Kim Y-S, Lim Y-J (2011) Primary stability and self-tapping blades: biomechanical assessment of dental implants in medium.density bone. Clin. Oral Impl. Res. 22, 1179-1184 DOI 10.1111/j.1600-0501.2010.01089.x
6. ASTM F543-00, Standard Specification and Test Methods for Metallic Medical Bone Screws, ASTM International, West Conshohocken, PA, 2002, at http://www.astm.org
7. ASTM F1839-08(2012), Standard Specification for Rigid Polyurethane Foam for Use as a Standard Material for Testing Orthopaedic Devices and Instruments, ASTM International, West Conshohocken, PA, 2012, at http://www.astm.org
8. Misch CE (2007) Contemporary implant dentistry. 3rd ed. Mosby Elsevier. St. Louis
9. Misch CE, Judy KW (1987) Classification of partially edentulous arches for implant dentistry. Int J Oral Implantol. 4(2):7-13.
10. Bardyn T, Gédet P, Hallermann W, Büchler P (2009) Quantifying the influence of bone density and thickness on resonance frequency analysis: an in vitro study of biomechanical test materials. Int J Oral Maxillofac Implants 24(6):1006-14
11. Sawbones at http://www.sawbones.com
12. Nagy P, Joób F. Á, Schindler Á, Pammer D, Bognár E (2014) Surface modification of dental implants. Biomechanica Hungarica 7(1):42-49
13. OsseoCare Pro at http://www.nobelbiocare.com

Author: David Pammer
Institute: Budapest University of Technology and Economics, Department of Materials Science and Engineering
Street: Bertalan Lajos utca 7
City: H-1111, Budapest
Country: Hungary
Email: pammer@eik.bme.hu

Effect of Arm Circumduction on Arterial Blood Flow

V. Szabó and G. Halász

Budapest University of Technology and Economics, Department of Hydrodynamic Systems,
1111 Budapest Műegyetem rkp. 3, Budapest, Hungary

Abstract— **Analyzing blood flow in a mobile arterial system is not an easy task. Our department has previously introduced a one dimensional model for the simulation of blood flow in static arterial systems using the method of characteristics [1] which has been modified by including the body acceleration caused by the inertial force into the momentum equation.**

The modified model was used to study the effect of periodic body acceleration, more specifically, arm circumduction on the arterial system. Exercises were performed with both arms symmetrically at three different levels of speed and three different angles. Average blood flow was calculated in the ascending aorta, the radial artery and the abdominal aorta.

As the results show, during arm circumduction blood flow increased in the radial artery and the ascending aorta. However, it slightly decreased in the abdominal aorta. The summarized description of the model and the limitations of the simulation are discussed in detail.

Keywords— **Artery system, momentum equation, blood flow, method of characteristics, body acceleration.**

I. INTRODUCTION

Blood flow analysis in a mobile human arterial system is a challenging task. Protocols for blood pressure measurement require patients to be motionless during the examination [2] [3]. Because of the difficulties to make measurement in a moving body, in order to study the effect of motion on blood flow, modeling is needed.

In the past several models were introduced to simulate pressure and flow propagation in a human arterial system. Some of them used lumped parameter methods e.g. the impedance method [4] [5] while others used distributed models e.g. the method of characteristics (MOC) [6] [7] [8] [9] or the two-step Lax-Wendroff method [10].

The effect of externally-imposed periodic body accelerations on blood flow in single arteries has also been studied previously [11], especially on blood flow in a stenosed artery [12] [13].

In a previous paper, we introduced a one dimensional model for the calculation of unsteady blood flow in the static arterial network using the method of characteristics [1]. In this present paper the modified version of this model is used to study the effect of body acceleration, particularly, arm circumduction on the blood flow in the mobile arterial system.

II. MODELS AND METHODS

The detailed description of the original model treating blood as a Newtonian fluid was published previously [1]. Here we summarize only the relevant information.

The arterial network of the model consists of 45 branches and is based on the schematic diagram of Avolio [4] (See Fig. 2). To take the viscoelasticity of the arterial vessels into account, the so called Stuart model was chosen (see Fig. 1), which is used for modeling viscoelasticity in polymertechnics [14]. In this model, the Kelvin-Voigt element (ε_2) represents viscoelastic deformation while the elastic spring element (ε_1) models the elastic deformation component. The viscoelastic material model was validated with several measurements carried out on a single silicone tube [15].

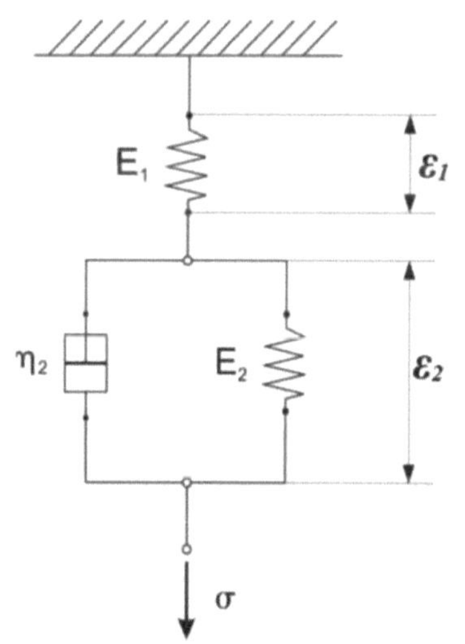

Fig. 1 Schematic diagram of the Stuart model (retrieved from [1])

Á. Jobbágy (ed.), *First European Biomedical Engineering Conference for Young Investigators*,
IFMBE Proceedings 50, DOI: 10.1007/978-981-287-573-0_22

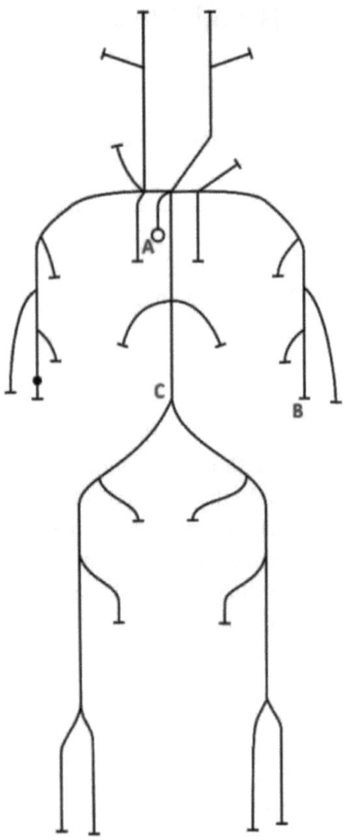

Fig. 2 Schematic diagram of the arterial system (adapted from [1])

Using the MOC as described in [16] and [17], the following system of partial differential equations are solved simultaneously:

1. Momentum equation:

$$\frac{\partial v}{\partial t}+v\frac{\partial v}{\partial x}+\frac{1}{\rho}\frac{\partial p}{\partial x}+g\frac{dh}{dx}+\frac{32\nu}{D^2}v=0 \quad (1)$$

2. Modified continuity equation:

$$2\frac{\partial \varepsilon}{\partial t}+2v\frac{\partial \varepsilon}{\partial x}+(2\varepsilon+1)\frac{\partial v}{\partial x}=0 \quad (2)$$

3. Equations of the Stuart model:

$$\frac{pD_0}{2\delta_0}(2\varepsilon+1)=E_1\varepsilon_1 \quad (3)$$

$$\frac{pD_0}{2\delta_0}(2\varepsilon+1)=E_2\varepsilon_2+\eta_2\dot{\varepsilon}_2 \quad (4)$$

$$\varepsilon=\varepsilon_1+\varepsilon_2 \quad (5)$$

where D_0 and D are the initial and instantaneous diameters, p transmural pressure, v axial velocity, h elevation, δ_0 wall thickness, ν kinematic viscosity, ε total deformation, g acceleration of gravity (9,81 m/s^2) and ρ density of the blood (1050 kg/m^3).

The parameters of the Stuart model (E_1, E_2 and η_2) are material properties of the vessel. In case of a single branch a simple genetic algorithm could be used to fine tune these parameters but since our model consists of 45 branches, the computational demands are far too high. Therefore the tuning of these parameters was performed on an empirical way.

Wave-propagation speed (a), diameter and strain are calculated using the Stuart model:

$$\varepsilon_2=\varepsilon_{2e}\cdot e^{-\frac{E_2}{\eta_2}\Delta t}+\frac{p_eD}{2\delta_0E_2}(2\varepsilon_e+1)\cdot\left(1-e^{-\frac{E_2}{\eta_2}\Delta t}\right) \quad (6)$$

$$\varepsilon=\varepsilon_2+\frac{p_eD}{2\delta_0E_1}(2\varepsilon_e+1) \quad (7)$$

$$a=\sqrt{\frac{E_1\delta_0}{\rho\,D_0}(\varepsilon+1)^{\frac{\beta}{2}}} \quad (8)$$

$$D=D_0(\varepsilon+1) \quad (9)$$

where ε_{2e} and ε_e are the viscoelastic and total deformation from the previous time step, p_e is the transmural pressure from the previous time step and Δt is the time step. In equation (8), the exponent β is chosen to be equal to 2 because in this case there is a linear correlation between the wave-speed (a) and the wall deformation (ε) which is in accordance with the observations of Anliker et al [18].

The arterioles and the capillaries were modeled using resistances with linear behavior:

$$\Delta p=R\cdot Q \quad (10)$$

where R and Q denotes the resistance and volume flow rate, respectively.

Equation (10) serves as a boundary condition on the outlet part. The periodic boundary condition at the inlet part (the heart) is given by the blood pressure graph throughout one heart cycle (see Fig. 3).

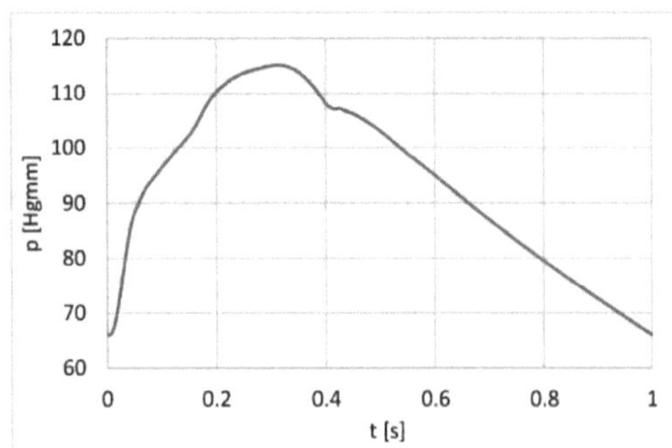

Fig. 3 Blood pressure at the heart

Setting proper initial conditions for each arterial branch and the interconnecting nodes is highly difficult. Therefore zero velocity, zero deformation and constant pressure was set. After starting the calculation the quasi-steady state is achieved within a few heart cycles.

In the original model, equation (1) is written in the relative coordinate system of the blood vessel, therefore only the parallel component of the acceleration caused by the gravitational force $\left(g\frac{dh}{dx}\right)$ is taken into account (that is, if the arterial branch is horizontal, it is omitted because $dh = 0$).

Since the force appearing in the momentum equation can be any function of position and time and the state of motion of the liquid [19], the application of the model can be extended from static to mobile arterial networks by including the body acceleration caused by the inertial force. Therefore, the modified version of equation (1) takes the following form:

$$\frac{\partial v}{\partial t} + v\frac{\partial v}{\partial x} + \frac{1}{\rho}\frac{\partial p}{\partial x} + g\frac{dh}{dx} + f_x + \frac{32\nu}{D^2}v = 0 \quad (11)$$

where f_x is the parallel component of the acceleration caused by the inertial force and depends on the time and the actual position of the artery.

Prior to applying the modified model on the whole arterial network, pressure distribution was calculated in a single rotating and accelerating tube. The numerical results matched well with the analytical solution which enabled us to use the new model for a more complex system.

The effect of arm circumduction on the human arterial system was studied in different cases. The exercise started from a horizontal position and was carried out symmetrically with both arms. The angular velocity (ω) and the aperture of the cone (α) described by the motion of the arms were different in each case. In each time step the parallel component of the total acceleration was calculated for each arterial branch based on their actual position. Values of pressure and velocity were computed by solving the equations defined previously. Finally, average blood flow was calculated in the ascending aorta, the radial artery and the abdominal aorta (points denoted by A, B, C on Fig. 2, respectively).

III. RESULTS

The results can be seen in Table 1(a)-(c). At given angle, blood flow rate increased in the ascending aorta and the radial artery as ω increased. At given angular velocity, blood flow decreased as α increased. However, in the first case ($\omega = 0.5$), the average blood flow slightly increased as α increased. We could demonstrate similar results for vessel segments located between the ascending aorta and the radial artery.

The difference between the average blood flow in the two wrists was negligible (<0.001 l/min). The behavior of the blood flow was the opposite in the abdomen. At given ω, the average blood flow increased with the increase of α. At given α, it decreased with the increase of ω.

Table 1. Average blood flow rates [l/min] in the heart (a), the left wrist (b) and the abdomen (c)

a)

	α=50°	α=100°	α=150°
$\omega = 0.5$	5.0277	5.0345	5.0433
$\omega = 1.0$	5.1315	5.1079	5.0713
$\omega = 1.5$	5.2044	5.1623	5.0976
$\omega = 2.0$	5.4091	5.3187	5.1664

b)

	α=50°	α=100°	α=150°
$\omega = 0.5$	0.0288	0.0288	0.0290
$\omega = 1.0$	0.0412	0.0376	0.0325
$\omega = 1.5$	0.0552	0.0475	0.0364
$\omega = 2.0$	0.0764	0.0630	0.0428

c)

	α=50°	α=100°	α=150°
$\omega = 0.5$	1.9621	1.9622	1.9622
$\omega = 1.0$	1.9622	1.9622	1.9623
$\omega = 1.5$	1.9597	1.9604	1.9614
$\omega = 2.0$	1.9570	1.9575	1.9588

IV. DISCUSSION

In this study an attempt was made to study the effect of motion on the blood flow in the human arterial system. In the model, the heart was assumed to have the same pressure distribution during the simulation. The viscoelastic parameters of the vessels as well as the peripheral resistance were constant too.

The study was limited to the arterial system without taking the effect of the venous blood flow into account. The deformation of the vessels caused by the motion and the surrounding muscles and other physiological effect were neglected too.

Although it is difficult to validate our results against in vivo data because of the large inter-personal variability and the methodological difficulties, the model presented above can be useful to make general observations on mobile arterial system and can help understand the effects of externally-imposed body acceleration on the blood flow.

Our results indicate that during arm circumduction blood flow increased in the vessels of the arms as well as in the heart. On the other hand, it decreased in the abdomen, which might suggest that arm circumduction augments blood flow in the moving body parts and impedes in the static ones.

The observation that blood flow increased parallel to the acceleration is similar to previous results for single arteries [20] [21].

However, because of limitations of the model and the lack of in vivo measurements, further studies need to be carried out in order to support this result.

V. CONCLUSION

In the present paper, a modified version of our previously published 1D model [1] for the simulation of blood flow in arterial system is presented which can be used to analyze blood flow in a moving arterial system.

To take the effect of motion into account, the body acceleration caused by the inertial force was included into the momentum equation and was calculated in each time step during the simulation based on the actual position of the arterial branch.

The model was used to study the effect of arm circumduction on the arterial system. Exercises were performed with both hands symmetrically at three different levels of speed and three different angles. Average blood flow was calculated in the heart, the left wrist and the abdomen.

During arm circumduction blood flow increased in the vessels of the arms as well as in the heart. On the other hand, it decreased in the abdomen, which might suggest that arm circumduction augments blood flow in moving body parts and impedes in static ones.

However, because of limitations of the model and the lack of in vivo measurements, further studies need to be carried out in order to support this result.

Conflict of Interest

The authors declare that they have no conflict of interest.

References

[1] G. Bárdossy and G. Halász, "Modeling blood flow in the arterial system," *Period. Polytech. Mech. Eng.*, vol. 55, no. 1, p. 49, May 2011.

[2] M. Mitka, "Many physician practices fall short on accurate blood pressure measurement.," *JAMA*, vol. 299, no. 24, pp. 2842–4, Jun. 2008.

[3] B. P. McGrath, "Ambulatory blood pressure monitoring.," *Med. J. Aust.*, vol. 176, no. 12, pp. 588–92, Jun. 2002.

[4] A. P. Avolio, "Multi-branched model of the human arterial system.," *Med. Biol. Eng. Comput.*, vol. 18, no. 6, pp. 709–718, 1980.

[5] N. Stergiopulos, D. F. Young, and T. R. Rogge, "Computer simulation of arterial flow with applications to arterial and aortic stenoses," *J. Biomech.*, vol. 25, no. 12, pp. 1477–1488, Dec. 1992.

[6] M. Anliker, R. L. Rockwell, and E. Ogden, "Nonlinear analysis of flow pulses and shock waves in arteries," *Zeitschrift für Angew. Math. und Phys. ZAMP*, vol. 22, no. 2, pp. 217–246, Mar. 1971.

[7] R. L. Rockwell, M. Anliker, and J. Elsner, "Model studies of the pressure and flow pulses in a viscoelastic arterial conduit," *J. Franklin Inst.*, vol. 297, no. 5, pp. 405–427, May 1974.

[8] J. C. Stettler, P. Niederer, and M. Anliker, "Theoretical analysis of arterial hemodynamics including the influence of bifurcations. Part I: mathematical models and prediction of normal pulse patterns.," *Ann. Biomed. Eng.*, vol. 9, no. 2, pp. 145–64, Jan. 1981.

[9] J. J. Wang and K. H. Parker, "Wave propagation in a model of the arterial circulation.," *J. Biomech.*, vol. 37, no. 4, pp. 457–70, Apr. 2004.

[10] K. Azer and C. S. Peskin, "A one-dimensional model of blood flow in arteries with friction and convection based on the Womersley velocity profile.," *Cardiovasc. Eng.*, vol. 7, no. 2, pp. 51–73, Jun. 2007.

[11] V. SUD and G. SEKHON, "Arterial flow under periodic body acceleration," *Bull. Math. Biol.*, vol. 47, no. 1, pp. 35–52, 1985.

[12] N. K. Verma, S. U. Siddiqui, and R. S. Gupta, "Pulsatile flow of blood in mild stenosis," *e-Journal Sci. Technol.*, vol. 6, no. 5, pp. 61–76, Feb. 2011.

[13] D. S. Sankar and U. Lee, "Nonlinear mathematical analysis for blood flow in a constricted artery under periodic body acceleration," *Commun. Nonlinear Sci. Numer. Simul.*, vol. 16, no. 11, pp. 4390–4402, Nov. 2011.

[14] G. Bodor and L. M. Vas, *Polymer Materials Science (in Hungarian)*. Műegyetemi Kiadó, 2000.

[15] G. Licskó and G. Bardossy, "Modelling blood flow in veins due to external pressure excitation," in *The 1st IMACS International Conference on Computational Biomechanics and Biology: Short communications*, 2007, p. ID256.

[16] V. L. Streeter and E. B. Wylie, *Hydraulic Transients*. New York, NY, USA: McGraw-Hill Book Company, 1967.

[17] J. Alastruey, K. H. Parker, J. Peiró, and S. J. Sherwin, "Analysing the pattern of pulse waves in arterial networks: a time-domain study," *J. Eng. Math.*, vol. 64, no. 4, pp. 331–351, Feb. 2009.

[18] M. Anliker, M. K. Wells, and E. Ogden, "The Transmission Characteristics of Large and Small Pressure Waves in the Abdominal vena Cava," *IEEE Trans. Biomed. Eng.*, vol. BME-16, no. 4, pp. 262–273, Oct. 1969.

[19] J. Serrin, *Mathematical principles of classical fluid mechanics*, vol. VIII. 1959, pp. 125 – 263.

[20] P. Nagarani and G. Sarojamma, "Effect of body acceleration on pulsatile flow of Casson fluid through a mild stenosed artery," *Korea-Australia Rheol. J.*, vol. 20, no. 4, pp. 189–196, 2008.

[21] M. El-Shahed, "Pulsatile flow of blood through a stenosed porous medium under periodic body acceleration," *Appl. Math. Comput.*, vol. 138, no. 2–3, pp. 479–488, Jun. 2003.

Author:	Viktor Szabó
Institute:	Budapest University of Technology and Economics, Faculty of Mechanical Engineering, Department of Hydrodynamic Systems
Street:	Műegyetem rkp. 3., D building, 3rd floor
City:	H-1111, Budapest
Country:	Hungary
Email:	vszabo@hds.bme.hu

Proposal of Alternative Thread Geometry for Use on Dental Implants

C. Ojeda[1], V. Chuman[2], and A. Arriola[2]

[1] Department of Mechanical and Electrical Engineering, Universidad de Piura (UDEP), Piura, Peru
[2] Cadillo de tecnologia S.A.C, Piura, Peru

Abstract— **With regard to the design of dental implants based on their geometrical characteristics and their influence on the mechanical behaviour of the implant and the response of the peri-implant bone, many pieces of research dealing with the matter can be found in the bibliography. Based on the observation of the geometrical parameters defined in such studies, one additional parameter was considered: the number of threads. After that, with the use of the Ansys Finite-Element-Analysis Software, three different commercial implants were analyzed and the results were taken as a basis for the proposal of a new design varying the geometrical parameter previously proposed. The result of the simulations show that this additional parameter should be taken into account when defining the geometry of the implant.**

Keywords— **Dental implants, Finite Element Analysis, Design.**

I. Introduction

There has been a significant amount of attempts to replicate dental pieces using alloplastic materials during recent years. Nevertheless, implant therapy based on scientific results appeared first with the results of the team directed by Dr. Branemark, giving definitive proof that pure titanium integrates with the osseous tissue if properly prepared[1]. Branemark's team proposed a threaded geometry to allow an easy adjustment of the implant[2].

After this discovery many implant systems have appeared on the market, offering implants with a wide variety of geometrics, sizes and surface treatments[1]. Nowadays, thanks to the availability of mechanical analysis software using the finite element method, the design process can be accelerated with simulated data of tissue behaviour, given the dificulty to obtain experimental data of the behaviour of living tissue[3, 4]. These simulated results must be validated with in-vitro and in-vivo clinical trials to ensure the feasibility and quality of the design.

There is a large amount of research that analyzes the behaviour of the osseo-implant system employing FEM tools, in which the selection of a representative section of the maxila to run the simulation on it can be observed, as well as different boundary condition assignments on said maxilla sections[5, 6, 7, 8, 9]. Different implant geometrical features have been taken into account to assess the behaviour of the implants analyzed in different studies and the influence of them on the peri-implant bone tissue[10, 11, 12].

The current work aims to compare the results obtained after simulating three different commercial implant geometries and one implant with the proposed geometry, all of them in one maxilla under the same loads and boundary conditions. The comparison is based on the strains, stresses and displacements on the implant and peri-implant bone tissue.

II. Material and Methods

A. Geometrical shape parameters

The analysis described in this paper is based on the shape parameters proposed separately by L. Baggi *et al.*[11], S. Desai *et al.* [12] and P. Ausiello *et al.* [10] and their findings.

L. Baggi *et al.*[11] define five shape parameter for their analysis, they are the fixture total length (L), the bone-implant interfacial length (l), the implant maximum diameter (d), the average thread pitch (p) and the average thread depth (t). S. Desai *et al.* [12] defines eight thread geometries leaving as constant the parameters L, l, d, p and t defined by Baggi. The different shapes proposed by Desai range from triangular and square to trapezoidal and buttress cross-sections. P. Ausiello *et al.* [10] define eight parameters, five of which are the same as the parameters defined by Baggi, while the other three are the thread width (w), the upper thread angle (α_1) and the lower thread angle (α_2), the upper thread angle being the one between a perpendicular to the implant axis and the thread surface that transfers most of the compressive load to the bone. The three works took into account a fully osseo-integrated system. Baggi and Ausiello worked with a 3D model, whereas S. Desai just developed a 2D analysis. Some of their conclusions are the following:

- The trapezoidal thread shape is the optimal thread cross-section shape for the reduction of stress and strain concentrations[12]. The optimal trapezoidal shape presented by S. Desai *et al.* [12] has an upper thread angle (α_1) and a lower thread angle (α_2) of 15° for both.

Á. Jobbágy (ed.), *First European Biomedical Engineering Conference for Young Investigators*,
IFMBE Proceedings 50, DOI: 10.1007/978-981-287-573-0_23

- The bone-implant interfacial length (l) barely affects the stress concentration on the cortical bone, but has a considerable influence on the stress concentration on the trabecular bone[11].
- The implant maximum diameter (d) has its main influence on the implant neck, i.e. on the cortical bone [11].
- The average thread pitch (p) is considered fundamental in achieving primary stability, where the maximum stress decreases when p decreases and l increases[10].
- The 0.8 mm pitch used by S. Desai *et al.* [12] is considered optimal by some references pointed out by P. Ausiello *et al.*[10].
- Results indicated that an optimal thread depth (t) and thread width (w) were 0.34 mm–0.5 mm and 0.18 mm–0.3 mm respectively[10].

P. Ausiello *et al.* [10] commented that in some of their references the implant pitch was considered of more importance in multiple-thread implants. However, the number of threads on the implant was not considered as a geometrical parameter by them.

Following the analysis of the results obtained in references [10, 11, 12] it could be seen that one of the parameters that had an important influence on the implant primary stability were the upper thread angle (α_1) and the lower thread angle (α_2). These parameters were taken into account only in one of the cited references, whereas the influence of these parameters can be regarded as a stress-strain transmission due to a wedge effect. Starting from the assumption of this wedge effect we could point out that the prior analysis just takes into account the upper and lower thread angles measured on a cross-section of the thread, but does not take into account the helix angle of the thread, which would be acceptable if the helix angle can be considered as a constant. In any other case, where the helix angle is not a constant, its influence can not be disregarded. In this case we could speak of a representative wedge angle, or a representative thread slope, which would modify the defined α_1 and α_2 to take into account the influence of the helix angle. This parameter has yet to be defined.

It can be noted that if the cases analyzed in [10, 11, 12] assume that all those implants have the same number of flutes on their threads, then the helix angle would be likely to be always the same. Nevertheless, if we consider multiple-thread implants, as mentioned by P. Ausiello *et al.* [10], the helix angle takes on a very important role in the stresses and strains produced due to this wedge effect on the peri-implant bone tissue.

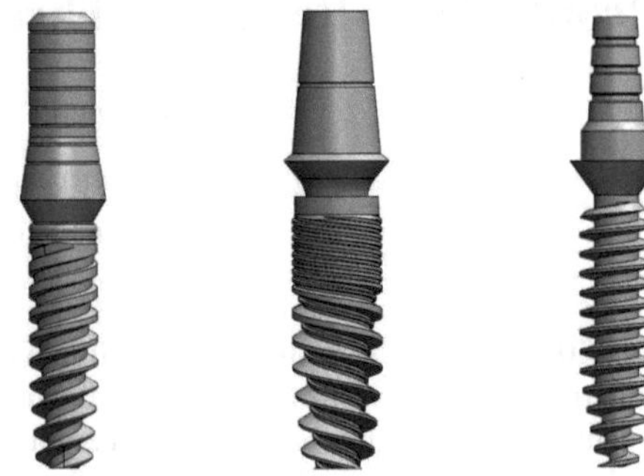

(a) Nova (b) Euroteknika (c) Odontit

Figure 1: Commercial implants taken as reference.

B. Commercial implant geometries

The commercial implant geometries were obtained using a profile projector for geometrical measurements and the SolidWorks software for the generation of the 3D geometry. All the geometries include the implant and abutment in one sole 3D solid, disregarding whether the original implant is a monoblock or not, which lately simplifies the analysis.

All the geometries obtained comply with the recommendation regarding the geometrical parameters stated in the previous subsection.

In the figure 1 the three different implants studied in this work are shown. The implant shown in fig. 1(a) represents a conical double thread implant from the Nova Implants company, while the one shown in fig. 1(b) represents a conical double thread implant with microthread on the implant neck from the Euroteknika company, and the implant shown in fig. 1(c) represents a cylindrical simple thread implant of the company Odontit.

Taking into account that the implants listed above are either double-threaded or single-threaded, a new triple-threaded implant (fig. 2) was proposed to evaluate the behaviour of such implant. The thread cross-section geometry of the proposed implant is based on that of the Nova implant with minor modifications. Later on the reason why will be clarified.

C. Mandible model

The model corresponding to the mandible to be simulated was generated from the CT images of a mandible using the segmentation and reverse engineering tools from the Mimics software. The modelled mandible corresponds to a 48-year-old patient, who conserved just 8 dental pieces and shows an important osseous resorption in the areas corresponding to the missing dental pieces. The properties of the trabecular

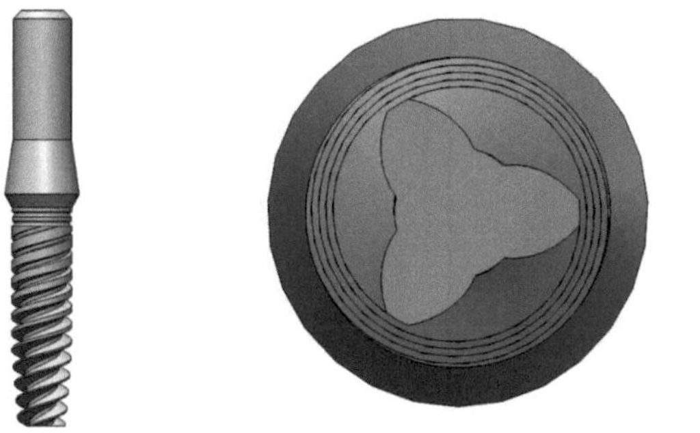

Figure 2: Proposed implant with triple thread

Table 1: Boundary and load conditions in the simulations

Implant	Boundary Conditions	Load Condition A	Load Condition B	Load Condition C
Nova	Fixed at both ends	324 N Oblique	314 N Vertical	100 N Oblique
Euroteknika	Fixed at both ends	324 N Oblique	314 N Vertical	100 N Oblique
Odontit	Fixed at both ends	324 N Oblique	314 N Vertical	100 N Oblique
Proposal	Fixed at both ends	324 N Oblique	314 N Vertical	100 N Oblique

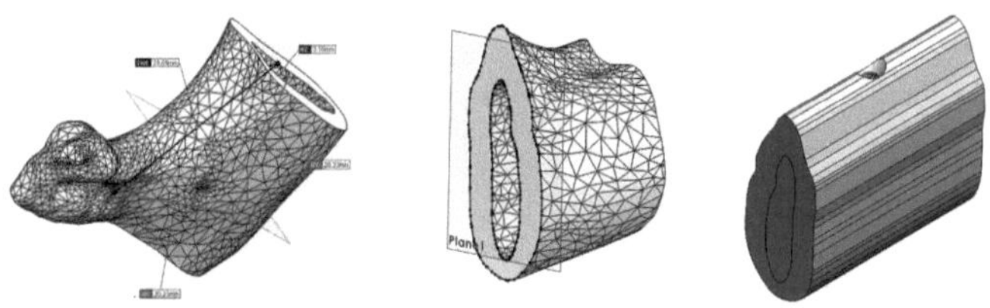

Figure 3: Mandible solid simplification

and cortical bone taken for the study correspond to the maximum of the values assigned to the different regions by a CT grayscale value function based on the relations presented by Rho et al. [13] and the Young modulus presented by Odin et al.[14]. The Young moduli assigned to the cortical and trabecular bone are respectively 16.28 MPa and 1.83 MPa. A Poisson number of 0.3 was considered in every analysis. All these values are close to those presented by Odin, Kayabasi and Mellal [5, 14, 7]. A simplified solid model for the mandible was obtained as an extrusion of the cross-sectional profile of the cortical and trabecular regions on the area where the implants were to be positioned, which can be seen in fig. 3.

D. Finite Element Model

The data related to boundary and load conditions presented by the different authors differ considerably, mainly due to the different masticatory conditions, patients' anatomies, patients' ages and peri-implant bone conditions, among others. The masticatory loads are not stable; they vary in magnitude and direction during mastication. In this process the implants are subject to different stress' distributions. In some cases, these distributions can lead to failure of the implant from marginal bone loss.[3].

Furthermore, it is necessary to select an appropriate mandible section in order to evaluate the effects of the implant on the peri-implant bone[15]. It is important to consider the mandible section where the effects of the loads on the implant are higher. These sections must be fixed with elastic restrictions to simulate the deformation of the rest of the mandible[15]. Nevertheless, the boundary load conditions are far from being specified with precision[3], this being the reason why there is a wide variety of assignments in the references consulted.

The loads used in this work have been taken from the data presented by Morneburg *et al.*[8] and is coherent with the data found in other references[9, 7, 5]. The different implants subject of the current work were analyzed applying the same boundary conditions and load conditions in all the cases. The proposed design is also included in the table. In every case, force and displacement convergence are pursued.

The load condition A (fig. 1) corresponds to the maximum load on the anterior area presented by Morneburg *et al.*[8] and the direction of the load follow that presented by O. Kayabasi *et al.* [7]. The load condition B resembles the one presented by Morneburg *et al.*[8] disregarding any inclination. The load condition C represents the medium load on the mandible anterior area presented by Morneburg *et al.*[8]. The influence of different friction coefficients was also taken into account for every case in order to analyze the pre-integration phase; the different friction coefficients will be seen further on in this work.

The software used for the analysis was Ansys v14.5. The mesh used was formed by tetrahedral solid elements and triangular contact elements (where applicable). For the different geometries, different meshes were used. To have an idea of the order of magnitude of the mesh size, an element count of around 60.000 and a node count of 100.000 can be taken as reference. For the configuration of the numerical model, the following conditions were defined: PURE PENALTY formulation, NODAL-NORMAL TO TARGET contact detection, contact stiffness of 0.01 and a stabilization damping factor of 0.35. General nonlinear force and displacement convergence

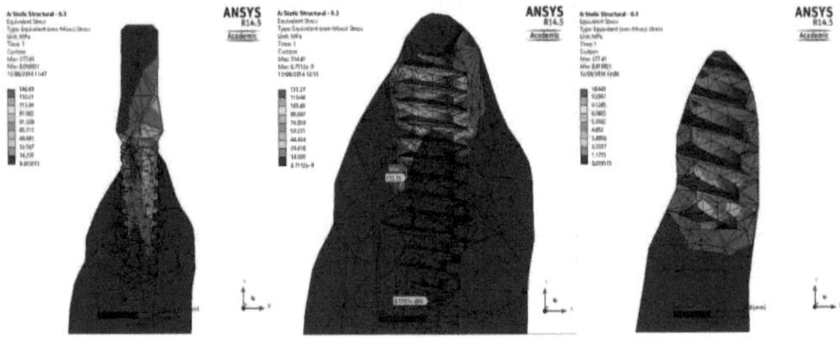

Figure 4: Von Mises stress distribution in the Nova implant with load condition A and 0.3 friction coefficient, showing maximum values in the implant (left), cortical bone (centre), and trabecular bone (right)

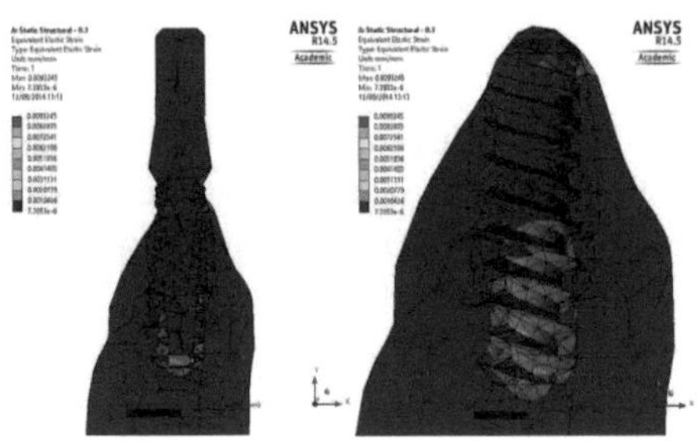

Figure 5: Von Mises strain distribution in the Nova implant with load condition A and 0.3 friction coefficient, showing maximum values in the implant (left) and bone tissue (right)

criteria of 0.5%, with a minimum reference of 0.01 N and 0.005 mm respectively: In both cases the convergence condition was auto-calculated by the solver on each substep. The LINE SEARCH option was activated to improve the convergence, and a constant stabilization with a damping factor of 0.35 was also applied from the first substep on. A stabilization force limit of 0.9 was also set.

III. RESULTS

The three commercial implants and the proposed one were simulated under the conditions described in the previous sections. From all the conditions listed in the table 1, the most critical is the load condition A with a friction coefficient of 0.3. In the figures 4 to 9, plots corresponding to these conditions for the three commercial implants can be seen. In fig. 11 and 12 the corresponding plots for the proposed design can be seen.

The relative displacements of the implant with respect to the peri-implant bone tissue were also taken into account for the assessment of the implant behaviour during the pre-integration phase. For load condition A and a 0.3 friction coefficient, the plots used to calculate the relative displacements on the commercial implants can be seen in fig. 10.

From fig. 10, relative displacements on the peri-implant

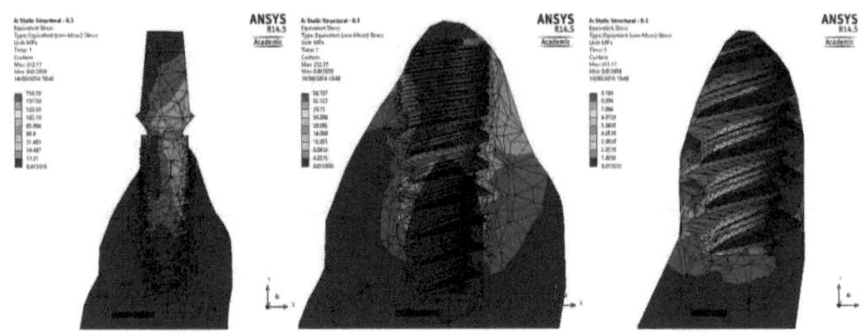

Figure 6: Von Mises stress distribution in the Euroteknika implant with load condition A and 0.3 friction coefficient, showing maximum values in the implant (left), cortical bone (centre), and trabecular bone (right)

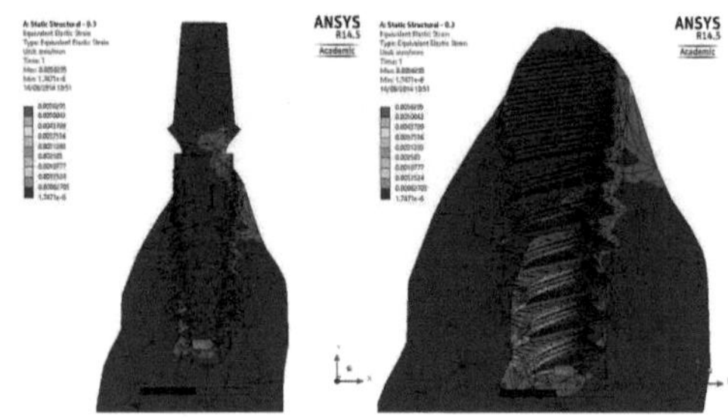

Figure 7: Von Mises strain distribution in the Euroteknika implant with load condition A and 0.3 friction coefficient, showing maximum values in the implant (left) and bone tissue (right)

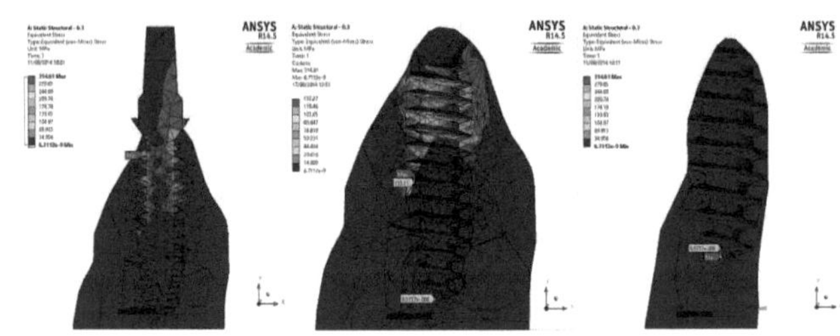

Figure 8: Von Mises stress distribution in the Odontit implant with load condition A and 0.3 friction coefficient, showing maximum values in the implant (left), cortical bone (centre), and trabecular bone (right)

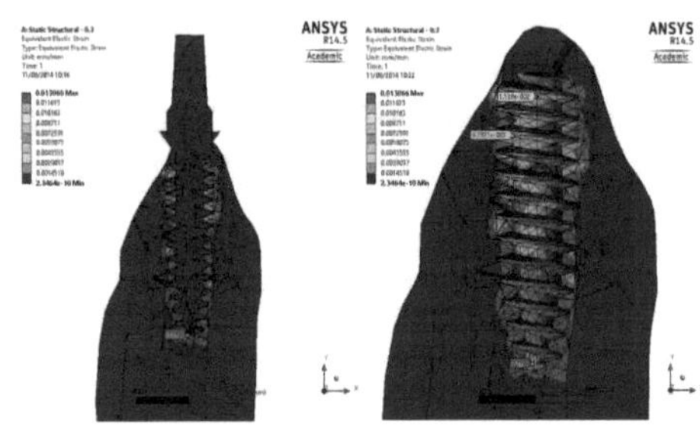

Figure 9: Von Mises strain distribution in the Odontit implant with load condition A and 0.3 friction coefficient, showing maximum values in the implant (left) and bone tissue (right)

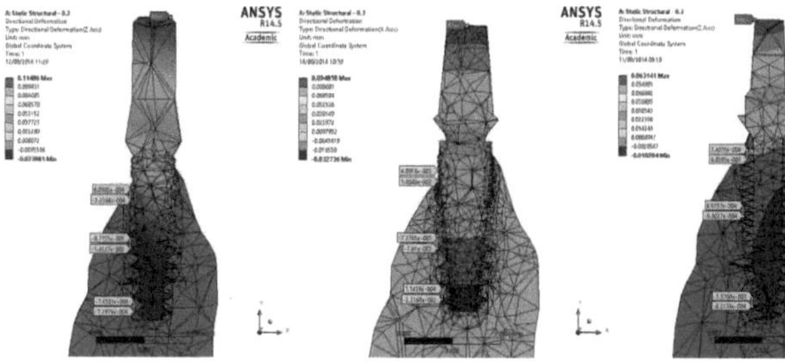

(a) Nova (b) Euroteknika (c) Odontit

Figure 10: Displacements in Z axis used to calculate the relative displacements

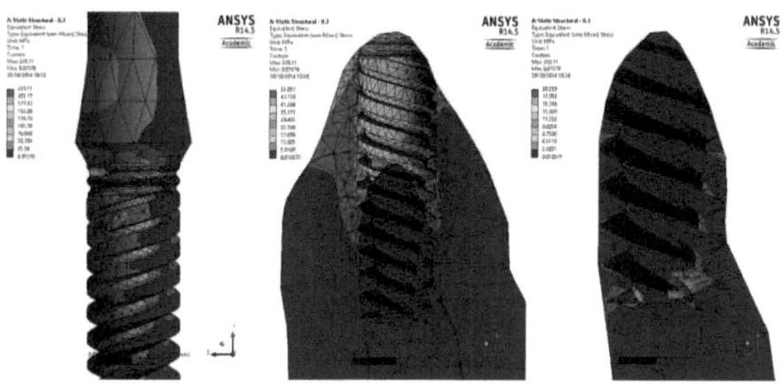

Figure 11: Von Mises stress distribution in the proposed implant with load condition A and 0.3 friction coefficient, showing maximum values in the implant (left), cortical bone (centre), and trabecular bone (right)

area of 0.00083 mm, 0.014 mm and 0.000086 mm respectively for the upper, middle, and lower thread regions of the Nova implant can be seen. For the Euroteknika implant, relative displacements on the peri-implant area of 0.01 mm, 0.0002 mm and 0.023 mm respectively for the upper, middle, and lower thread regions can be seen. For the Odontit implant, relative displacements on the peri-implant area of 0.00729 mm, 0.0013 mm and 0.0049 mm respectively for the upper, middle, and lower thread regions can be seen. The displacement convergence criteria for the Nova, Euroteknika and Odontit cases is 3.38E-06, 1E-03 and 5.81E-05 respectively. If the relative displacements calculated are too close to these values, the ony conclusion that can be reached from them is that the relative displacements are negligible.

The table 2 summarizes the results obtained for the different conditions in the different implants. With the help of this table it can be clarified that the cross-sectional thread profile of the Nova implant was taken as reference to model the triple-threaded implant because of its simplicity and good behaviour in most cases.

IV. Discussion

1. It can be observed that there is always a better stress and strain distribution with full osseo-integrated implants.

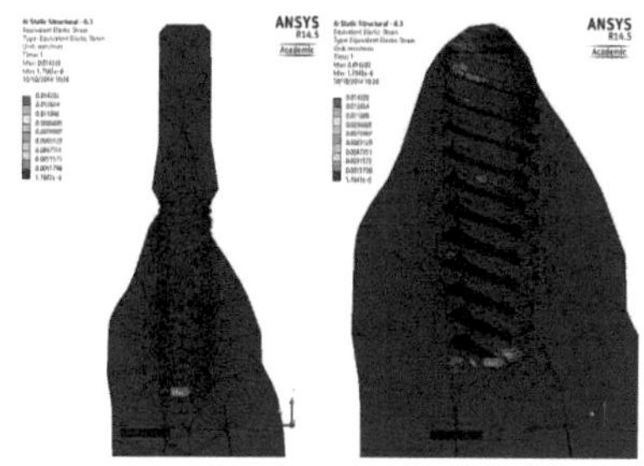

Figure 12: Von Mises strain distribution in the Odontit implant with load condition A and 0.3 friction coefficient, showing maximum values in the implant (left) and bone tissue (right)

2. The Nova implant present the lowest stresses in most cases followed by the Euroteknika, both double-threaded implants. Both are better than the Odontit, a single-threaded implant, in all of the cases except those where there is a full osseo-integration, where the Odontit implant presents the lowest stresses.
3. Taking as reference the yield strengh of the cortical bone as 115 MPa [16] and that of the trabecular bone as 5 MPa[6], the Odontit implant present a very low stress concentration on the trabecular bone for all cases while, on the other hand, a very high stress concentration on the cortical bone in the pre-integration phase is present. On its side, the Euroteknika and Nova present a better distribution. In cases of oblique load with friction, the Euroteknika is the one with the better behaviour, always keeping the stresses at the post-integration below both bone yield strengths. The Nova implant does not present such good behaviour on the trabecular bone, where it shows stresses higher than those permissible.
4. If a fatigue yield strength of 30 MPa for 10E06 cycles is also taken into account [16], it can be seen that complete integration cases present stresses bellow this limit. During the integration phase of 6 to 8 months [2] it is very unlikely to reach such a number of load cycles as to lead the system to failure.
5. The strains are always under the normal maximum values for human bone tissue.
6. The three commercial implants analyzed present relative displacements of the order of hundredths of a millimeter. In the case of the Nova implant they could be even negligible.
7. For full osseo-integration, the proposed implant presents similar stresses to the commercial implants analyzed, but almost always higher values. In any case, they are not high enough to lead to a system failure.
8. Taking as reference the yield strength of the cortical bone as 115 MPa [16] and that of the trabecular bone as 5

Table 2: Summary of the results obtained

Implant	Load(N)	Friction Coeffi-cient	Max. Relative Displace-ment(mm)	Displacement Convergence Criteria	Max. Stress on Assem-bly(MPa)	Max. Stress on Corti-cal(MPa)	Max. Stress on Trabecu-lar(MPa)	Max. Strain on Assemby	Max. Strain on bone
Nova	324 Oblique	0.3	0.014	3.38E-006	146.49	35.96	10.44	0.009	0.009
Nova	324 Oblique	1	0.002	1.00E-006	300.09	50.4	14.975	0.013	0.013
Nova	324 Oblique	Bonded	-	-	269.5	23.175	14.975	0.0036	0.0036
Nova	314 Vertical	0.3	0.000008	4.35E-006	128.27	26.715	10.207	0.00995	0.00995
Nova	314 Vertical	Bonded	-	-	74.264	16.684	3.203	0.0036	0.0036
Nova	100 Oblique	0.3	0.000024	1.26E-006	106.73	29.67	11.64	0.0175	0.0175
Nova	100 Oblique	Bonded	-	-	85.76	7.59	1.2795	0.00225	0.00225
Euroteknika	324 Oblique	0.3	0.023	1.00E-003	154.78	36.137	9.104	0.0056	0.0056
Euroteknika	324 Oblique	1	0.01	1.00E-003	154.64	38.3	8.47	0.0057	0.0057
Euroteknika	324 Oblique	Bonded	-	-	212.49	31.937	3.3855	0.0025	0.0025
Euroteknika	314 Vertical	0.3	0.0014	1.00E-003	59.228	27.45	4.397	0.0045	0.0045
Euroteknika	314 Vertical	Bonded	-	-	58.54	15.368	3.55	0.002	0.002
Euroteknika	100 Oblique	0.3	0.0079	1.00E-003	67.525	12.654	3.83	0.0028	0.0028
Euroteknika	100 Oblique	Bonded	-	-	67.61	10.116	1.083	0.0019	0.0019
Odontit	324 Oblicua	0.3	0.0073	5.81E-005	314.61	133.27	0.0000085	0.013	0.013
Odontit	324 Oblique	1	0.0048	2.05E-004	372.15	127.62	0.000015	0.0137	0.0137
Odontit	324 Oblique	Bonded	-	-	214.88	20.887	0.000005	0.003	0.003
Odontit	314 Vertical	0.3	0.0046	2.50E-005	285.73	134.33	0.000004	0.037	0.0137
Odontit	314 Vertical	Bonded	-	-	82.72	13.545	0.000006	0.00315	0.00315
Odontit	100 Oblique	0.3	0.0044	3.49E-005	292.78	139.39	0.000005	0.012	0.012
Odontit	100 Oblique	Bonded	-	-	68.39	8.77	0.0000001	0.00098	0.00098
Proposal	324 Oblique	0.3	0.02	1.00E-004	228.11	53.051	20.239	0.0142	0.0142
Proposal	324 Oblique	1	0.007	1.00E-004	237.81	67.382	27.899	0.0195	0.0195
Proposal	324 Oblique	Bonded	-	-	238.91	41.408	2.8278	0.0026	0.0026
Proposal	314 Vertical	0.3	0.0052	1.00E-004	71.105	61.688	20.303	0.01423	0.01423
Proposal	314 Vertical	Bonded	-	-	79.939	14.901	3.1004	0.00177	0.00177
Proposal	100 Oblique	0.3	0.0059	1.00E-004	72.822	57.14	18.72	0.01363	0.01363
Proposal	100 Oblique	Bonded	-	-	76.024	13.177	0.90071	0.00082	0.00082

MPa[6], the proposed implant shows permissible stresses for all the cases at a post-integration phase. This behaviour equals that of the Euroteknika and improves the behaviour of the Nova.

9. For the fatigue assumption described in point 4, it is also very unlikely for the proposed implant to reach such a number of load cycles as to lead the system to failure.
10. In the proposed implant, the strains are also always under the normal maximum values for human bone tissue.
11. For the proposed implant, the relative displacements are very low as well, and most of the times can be neglected.
12. If we concentrate on the 100 N oblique load, considering it as the normal condition of low load for the pre-integration phase, the Euroteknika is the only one that does not surpass the yield strengths for both bones.

V. Conclusion

From the discussed observations the following conclusions can be reached:

1. The good behaviour of the Nova and Euroteknika implants, as well as the proposed triple-threaded implant, suggest that a multiple thread could be a beneficial geometry for use in implant designs in contrast to the single-threaded geometry.
2. The microthread, present in the Euroteknika implant, contributes to a reduction of the stress concentration, mainly during the pre-integration phase.
3. Despite not being better than either the Euroteknika or the Nova implants in the preintegration phase, the proposed implant outranges the Nova implant in the postintegration phase, having a very low stress for a 324 N oblique load in comparison with the stress presented by the Nova implant. This shows the possible beneficial effects of a triple-threaded implant.

It should also be pointed out that no rigorous method was used to define the triple-threaded implant geometry, and yet it presented benefits when compared with the Nova implant. It is recommended to further study implants with thread numbers higher than 2 in order to have a picture of their possible benefits on implant designs.

It is also recommended to study a triple-threaded implant with microthread, as the addition of the microthread feature could overcome some of the weaknesses that the proposed implant still has.

Acknowledgment

The authors would like to thank the innovation fund Fondo para la Innovacion, Ciencia y Tecnologia (FINCyT) (N° 215- FINCYT-IB-2013) for providing the research grant to finance the current work.

References

1. Jokstad A, Braegger U, Brunski J et al. Quality of dental implants. *Int Dent J.* 2003;53:409–443.
2. Branemark P. Introduction to Osseointegration in *Tissue-Integrated Prostheses*:51–56.Quintessence Publishing 1985.
3. Soncini M, Pietrabissa R, Natali A et al. Testing the reliability of dental implant devices in *Dental Biomechanics* (Natali A. , ed.):111–127.Taylor & Francis 2003.
4. Spiekermann H, Donath K, Hassel T et al. Biomechanics in *Color Atlas of Dental Medicine: Implantology* (Rateitschak K, Wolf H. , eds.):81–90.Georg Thieme Verlag 1994.
5. Mellal A, Wiskott H, Botsis J et al. Stimulating effect of implant loading on surrounding bone. Comparison of three numerical models and validation by in vivo data. *Clin Oral Implants Res.* 2004;15:239–248.
6. Garitaonaindia U, Alcaraz J. Análisis mediante simulación numérica de implantes dentales con microrosca in *XVIII Congreso nacional de ingeniería mecánica, Asociación española de ingeniería mecánica*;1:1–8 2010.
7. Kayabasi O, Yüzbasioglu E, Erincanli F. Static, dynamic and fatigue behaviors of dental implant using finite element method. *Advances in Engineering Software.* 2006;37:649–658.
8. Morneburg T, Pröschel P. Measurements of masticatory forces and implant loads: a methodologic study. *Int J Prosthodont.* 2002;15(1):20–7.
9. Field C, Li Q, Li W et al. Influence of tooth removal on mandibular bone response to mastication. *Arch Oral Biol.* 2008;53:1129–1137.
10. Ausiello P, Franciosa P, Martorelli M et al. Effects of thread features in osseo-integrated titanium implants using a statistics-based finite element method. *Dent Mater.* 2012;28:919–927.
11. Baggi L, Cappelloni I, Maceri F et al. Stress-based performance evaluation of osseointegrated dental implants by finite-element simulation. *Simulation Modelling Practice and Theory.* 2008;16:971–987.
12. Desai S, Desai M, Katti G et al. Evaluation of design parameters of eigth dental implant designs: A two-dimensional finite element analysis. *Nigerian Journal of Clinical Practice.* 2012;15(2):176–181.
13. Rho J, Hobatho M, Ashman R. Relations of mechanical properties to density and CT numbers in human bone. *Med Eng Phys.* 1995;17(5):347–355.
14. Odin G, Savoldelli C, Bouchard P et al. Determination of Young's modulus of mandibular bone using inverse analysis. *Med Eng Phys.* 2010;32(6):630–637.
15. Natali A, Pavan P. Numerical approach to dental biomechanics in *Dental Biomechanics* (Natali A. , ed.):211–238.Taylor & Francis 2003.
16. Natali A, Hart R, Pavan P et al. Mechanics of bone tissue in *Dental Biomechanics* (Natali Arturo N.. , ed.):1–17.Taylor & Francis 2003.
17. Ayllón J. Informe sobre ensayos de fatiga deimplantes dedental endoóseos tipo SURGIMPLANT CE gr IV de la empresa Galimplant S.L. tech. rep. Laboratotio de Ingeniería Mecánica, Escuela superior de Ingenieros, Universidad de Sevilla 2012.
18. Bonollo F, Natali A, Pavan P. Dental devices in titanium-based materials via casting route in *Dental Biomechanics* (Natali A. , ed.):90–109.Taylor & Francis 2003.
19. Branemark P, Engstrand P, Nannmark U et al. Branemark Novum: Prosthodontic and Dental Laboratory Procedures for Fabrication of a Fixed Prothesis on the Day of Surgery. *Int J Prosthodont.* 2001;14:303–309.

20. Cano D. Determinación de piezas dentarias perdidas y brechas edéntulas a restaurar en una población adulta de trabajadores de una empresa petrolera de la provincia de talara en el año 2009. Master's thesis Facultad de Estomatología Roberto Beltrán, Universidad Peruana Cayetano Heredia 2010.
21. Choi K, Goldstein S. A comparison of the fatigue behavior of human trabecular and cortical bone Tissue. *J Biomech.* 1992;25(12):1371–1381.
22. Chuman V. Diseño y simulación de implantes dentales. Primer Informe: Estado del arte. tech. rep. Universidad de Piura 2014.
23. Chuman V. Diseño y simulación de implantes dentales. Informe Final: Modelamiento y simulación de implantes comerciales - Propuesta de implante propio. tech. rep. Universidad de Piura 2014.
24. Chuman V. Estudio computacional de implantes dentales. Primer Informe: Simulación de implantes propios UDEP. tech. rep. Universidad de Piura 2014.
25. Colauto E. Desenvolvimento de Pino intra-radicular, resistência à fratura e análise da distribução de tensões a través do método dos elementos finitos. Master's thesis Facultade de Odontología de São José dos Campos, Universidade Estadual Paulista 2008.
26. Coutinho T, Ferrás P, Sampaio J et al. The biomechanical model challenge with angled implants in *Proc, I Int Conf on Biodent Eng*;1:177–179. 2009.
27. Fernández E, Gil F, Aparicio C et al. Materials in implantology in *Dental Biomechanics* (Natali A. , ed.):69–87.Taylor & Francis 2003.
28. Gil F, Aparicio A Crespo C et al. Aflojamiento de tornillos de conexión implante dental - prótesis mediante simulación de cargas cíclicas masticatorias. *Anales de mecánica de la fractura.* 2003;20:491–494.
29. Gröning F, Fagan M, O'Higgins P. Modeling the human mandible under masticatory loads: Which input variables are important? *The anatomical record.* 2012;295:853–863.
30. Hunter R, Alister F, Möller J et al. Develop mono-block tooth implants using automate design and FEM analysis. *Archives of Materials Science and Engineering.* 2007;28:261–268.
31. Ikeda M, Ceccarelli J, Proaño D. Periimplantitis y mucositis periimplantaria. *Revista Estomatológica Herediana.* 2007;17(2):90–98.
32. Korioth T, Hannam A. Deformation of the human mandible during simulated tooth clenching. *J Dent Res.* 1994;73(1):56–66.
33. Lemus L, Almagro Z, León C. Origen y evolución de los implantes dentales. *Revista Habanera de Ciencias Médicas [Online].* 2009;8(4):Retrieved from ¡http://www.redalyc.org/articulo.oa?id=180414045030¿. Accessed 07 Aug 2012.
34. Natali A, Pavan P, Meroi E. Mechanics of materials in *Dental Biomechanics* (Natali A. , ed.):240–264.Taylor & Francis 2003.
35. Office of device evaluation, Dental device branch . Special Controls Guidance Document: Root-form Endosseous Dental Implants and Endosseous Dental Abutments. 2004.
36. Ojeda C, Arriola A, Chuman V et al. Validación de modelos anatómicos virtuales de mandíbulas de pacientes peruanos para el estudio en el diseño de implantes dentales. Manuscript presented to Universidad de Piura in the framework of the project 215-FINCyT-IA-2013.
37. Ojeda C, Chuman V, Arriola A. Influence of the selection of the boundary conditions and analysis region on the results of dental implants FEM simulation. Paper presented at the VII Conference on Biomedical Engineering at the Universidad de Concepción, Chile, 3–4 November 2014.
38. Ojeda J, Martinez-Reina J, Mayo J.. Simulation of the behaviour of mandibular periimplant bone with a remodeling model in *Proc, I Int. Conf. on Biodent. Eng.*;1:23–27 2009.
39. Ozeki K, Fukui Y, Aoki H. Hydroxyapatite Coated Dental Implants by Sputtering Technique. *Biocybernetics & Biomed Eng.* 2006;26(1):95–101.
40. Pérez M, García-Aznar J, Doblaré M et al. A mechanobiological model for bone ingrowth on dental implants in *Proc, I Int Conf on Biodent Eng*;1:89–93 2009.
41. Pi Urgell J, Vericat Queralt J. Branemark Novum: una alternativa para la rehabilitación del maxilar superior desdentado. *RCOE.* 2002;7:21–28.
42. Tauber M. Puesta al día: Prótesis con implantes *Quintessence técnica (ed. esp).* 2007;19(2):85–91.
43. Vanegas J, Landinez N, Garzón-Alvarado D. A numerical framework for wound healing at the bone-dental implant interface in *Proc, I Int. Conf. on Biodent. Eng.*;1:145–151 2009.
44. van Oosterwyck H, van der Sloten J, Duyck J et al. Computer-aided, pre-surgical analysis for oral rehabilitation in *Dental Biomechanics* (Natali A. , ed.):52–67.Taylor & Francis 2003.

Author: Carlos Ojeda
Institute: Universidad de Piura
Street: Av. Ramon Mugica 131
City: Piura
Country: Peru
Email: carlos.ojeda@udep.pe

Novel, Inverse Biomechanical Methods Supporting Abdominal Aortic Aneurysm Management

Róbert Nagy and Imre Bojtár

Department of Structural Mechanics, Budapest University of Technology and Economics, Budapest, Hungary

Abstract— **Clinical treatment of abdominal aortic aneurysms is decided mainly on the maximal dilatation diameter. Biomechanics based criteria calculated by numerical fluid structure interaction simulations on patient specific geometries are superior to that approach, but are extremely time and resource consuming and require high expertise, furthermore they fail to incorporate the real, inhomogenous material parameters. Our method, summarized in this paper, handles these shortcomings by introducing a novel, indirect, in-vivo, patient-specific inverse material parameter identification method.**

Keywords— **abdominal aortic aneurysm, rupture risk, material parameters, ECG-gated CTA, inverse isogeometric FEM**

I. INTRODUCTION

A. Abdominal aortic aneurysms

Abdominal aneurysm is an irreversible local dilatation of the aorta. The healthy diameter range of an aorta is from 15 mm to 24 mm [1]. Aneurysm is diagnosed when it exceeds 30 mm [2, 3]. If bigger than 55 mm, it is called large aneurysm; below it is classified as small. The mortality ratio of their ensuing rupture is over 80% [4, 5], a disturbing stagnating figure in the last decades. This fact, along with the prevalence ratio in the population above 50 [6, 7] poses a serious burden on the healthcare system.

B. Treatment

The advent of regular screening tests (ultrasound and X-ray) enabled early recognition and consequent elective open surgery or endovascular grafting [8], procedures still retaining significant mortality and morbidity rates, thus it is vital to separate dilatations highly prone to rupture from stable ones. A strong positive correlation was observed between the maximal diameter of the dilatation an probability of rupture [9], which can be explained on mechanical grounds by Laplace's law of thin curved membranes. Current consensus states that the rupture risk grows higher than the mortality of elective surgery among large aneurysms, and clinical practice also relies mainly on this criterion (large aneurysms are treated by surgery, small ones are followed up).

II. MOTIVATION

A. State-of-the-art

Insufficient operative effectiveness [10] and the still occurring rupture of small aneurysms demanded an improved decision strategy based on biomechanical concepts: rupture occurs when the pulsating blood flow induced stresses in the vessel wall exceed the tissue's limit strength. Patient specific numerical modeling adopting this concept was proven to be superior to the maximal diameter [11] with good reproducibility [12].

In most cases the partial differential equations describing the fluid and solid phases are handled separately in an arbitrary Lagrangian-Eulerian (ALE) description by the best suited finite volume (FV) and finite element (FE) methods, respectively and are fully coupled together in a fluid-structure interaction (FSI) procedure. The geometry is obtained by modalities such as computer tomography (CT) or magnetic resonance (MR) at a single instant of time; the pressure and the volumetric flow rate profile is measured at the arm and then transformed by a one dimensional model of the arterial system [13] to transient boundary conditions of the fluid phase at the arterial section of interest. Implementing a proper non-Newtonian material model for the blood, the CFD calculation results in the pressure field, the boundary condition of the hyperelastic or viscoelastic solid model, which itself is embedded in an elastic support environment. On the other hand, the displacement field, the result of the FE simulation serves as the boundary condition of the CFD run. This concept requires an iteration algorithm in each timestep of the unsteady problem until the dynamic equilibrium is fulfilled.

B. Pitfalls

One of the greatest shortcomings of this framework is the fact, that the distribution of the material parameters is unknown, however it is observed to vary up to an order of magnitude even in the same person due to the degradation process [14, 15], underestimating the stress concentration on the

Á. Jobbágy (ed.), *First European Biomedical Engineering Conference for Young Investigators*,
IFMBE Proceedings 50, DOI: 10.1007/978-981-287-573-0_24

one hand and overestimating the resistance of the tissue on the other.

III. PURPOSE

Our intention is to develop a new, non invasive method to measure the in-vivo material parameters of the tissue [16]. This way we amend the stress calculations, complete our understanding of tissue degradation throughout the inflation of the lumen and provide a better basis for management decisions.

IV. NUMERICAL METHOD

A. Imaging modality

Exploiting the new possibilities of the latest imaging techniques [17], we adopt the electrocardiogram gated computed tomography angiography (ECG-gated CTA) – commonly used in case of the heart – for the aorta, with which instead of having only one geometry at a single instance of time, we gain new insights into its dynamic behavior. We used a Philips Brilliance iCT (Koninklijke Philips NV, Best, Netherlands) device, and captured the shape of the lumen in ten equal timesteps of a heartbeat; the spatial resolution is approximately 0.5 mm in the transverse and 1 mm in the axial directions respectively. Finally, the surface of the lumen at the timesteps is acquired by an active contour algorithm.

B. Displacement field

The above described geometry moving in time does not contain the displacement field since the nodes are not connected. To solve this problem artificial makers or natural landmark tracking could be used, but these methods either necessitate sophisticated experimental setup or are highly invasive, and we want to avoid both. The displacement determination solely from our data is an ill-posed problem, and can be solved by incorporating it in the final weak formulation or imposing certain constraints. We followed this latter path to be able to detach the load calculation from the final iteration of the material parameters. Based on previous FSI simulations, we hypothesized the incremental displacement to coincide with the corresponding corrected surface normal. The correction is the constraint of the periodic movement, which also serves as the measure of the goodness of the hypothesis. By increasing the temporal resolution the correction term vanishes.

C. Isogeometric analysis

We determine a parametric two dimensional bicubic spline representation of the lumen surface, which is also used to mitigate the measurement errors of the nodal positions. After a projection algorithm, exploiting the affine covariance of splines, we describe only the movement of the knots by trigonometric series, this way representing the lumen motion function. Recent trends in FE analysis turned towards using the functions describing the geometry as basis functions for the numerical model as well, evading the meshing process and enabling the work on the exact geometry [18, 19]. We also use this principle, with which it is also easier to provide the necessary continuity conditions for the novel isochor Kirchhoff shell element we introduced as a modification of the general Cosserat theory.

D. Fluid simulation

The FSI iteration is the most time and resource consuming part of the usual approach. We avoid it by taking advantage of the known wall motion function and use it as a moving boundary condition in a simple fluid simulation.

E. Material parameter identification

The resulting displacement and load fields are the two pillars of the final material parameter identification process. The power of the flow induced forces should be equal to the time derivative of the sum of the strain energy and kinetic energy of the wall. The power is calculated from the loads and the reference surface velocity function. The kinetic energy is given by the shell model and the reference surface velocity function, while for the estimate of strain energy we need additional characteristics of the material model, for which well developed formulas are in the literature based on a microstructural approach [20]. Model parameter identification was carried out by a fast Levenberg-Marquardt local optimization algorithm where the objective function gradient is provided numerically in time comparable to a normal function evaluation by virtue of the local support property of the spline basis functions.

V. EXPERIMENTAL VALIDATION

Aneurysmal aortic sections were dissected from patients undergoing open surgery at the Heart and Vascular Center of Semmelweis University, where the ECG-gated CTA images were also taken preceding the operations.

A. Macroscopic behavior

We measured macroscopic elastic behavior of the specimens by using displacement controlled equi-biaxial tensile tests at the laboratory of Semmelweis University, Institute of Human Physiology and Clinical Experimental Research to match the calculated result.

B. Microstructure

At Semmelweis University, Department of Biophysics and Radiation Biology the microstructure of the same samples was assessed by multi-photon microscopy, which is capable to visualize collagen throughout the cross-section of arterial constitutive layers. We stacked image slices together in order to get 3D data, and by the aid of an automatic image processing algorithm we were able to determine the collagen content and the distribution function of the fiber orientation by applying a 3D Fourier transform.

VI. CONCLUSIONS

With the presented procedure we are able to capture the dynamic behavior of the arterial wall, deduce the distribution of the hyperelastic material model associated with it. As a result we can quantify calcification of the aging artery, highlight the damaged area of aneurysms and compare them to the healthy tissue in the same patient.

CONFLICT OF INTEREST

The authors declare that they have no conflict of interest.

REFERENCES

1. Liddington M. I., Heather B. P.. The relationship between aortic diameter and body habitus *European Journal of Vascular Surgery.* 1992;6:89-92.
2. McGregor J. C., Pollock J. G., Anton H. C.. The value of ultrasonography in the diagnosis of abdominal aortic aneurysm *Scottish Medical Journal.* 1975;20:133-137.
3. Johnston K. W., Rutherford R. B., Tilson M. D., Shah D. M., Hollier L., Stanley J. C.. Suggested standards for reporting on arterial aneurysms. Subcommittee on Reporting Standards for Arterial Aneurysms, Ad Hoc Committee on Reporting Standards, Society for Vascular Surgery and North American Chapter, International Society for Cardiovascular Surgery *Journal of Vascular Surgery.* 1991;13:452-58.
4. Ingoldby C. J., Wujanto R., Mitchell J. E., Epstein D. M., Sculpher M. J., Greenhalgh R. M.. Impact of vascular surgery on community mortality from ruptured aortic aneurysms *The British Journal of Surgery.* 1986;360:551-553.
5. Kantonen Ilkka, Lepäntalo Mauri, Brommels Mats, et al. Mortality in ruptured abdominal aortic aneurysms *European journal of vascular and endovascular surgery.* 1999;17:208–212.
6. Lederle F. A., Johnson G. R., Wilson S. E., al. . The aneurysm detection and management study screening program: Validation cohort and final results *Archives of Internal Medicine.* 2000;160:1425-1430.
7. Lederle F. A., Johnson G. R., Wilson S. E.. Abdominal aortic aneurysm in women *Journal of Vascular Surgery.* 2001;34:122-126.
8. Brown L.C., Powell J.T., Thompson S.G.. The UK EndoVascular Aneurysm Repair (EVAR) trials: randomised trials of EVAR versus standard therapy *Health Technology Assessment.* 2012;16:1-218.
9. Szilagyi D Emerick, Smith Roger F, DeRusso Franklin J, Elliott Josei'h P, Sherrin Frederick W. Contribution of abdominal aortic aneurysmectomy to prolongation of life. *Annals of Surgery.* 1966;164:678.
10. Powell J.T.. Final 12-year follow-up of Surgery versus Surveillance in the UK Small Aneurysm Trial *British Journal of Surgery.* 2007;94:702–708.
11. Fillinger M. F., Marra S. P., Raghavan M. L., Kennedy F. E.. Prediction of rupture risk in abdominal aortic aneurysm during observation: Wall stress versus diameter *Journal of Vascular Surgery.* 2003;37:724-732.
12. Hyhlik-Dürr Alexander, Krieger Tim, Geisbüsch Philipp, Kotelis Drosos, Able Thomas, Böckler Dittmar. Reproducibility of deriving parameters of AAA rupture risk from patient-specific 3D finite element models *Journal of Endovascular Therapy.* 2011;18:289–298.
13. Bárdossy Gergely, Halász Gábor. Modeling blood flow in the arterial system *Mechanical Engineering.* 2012;55:49–55.
14. Speelman Lambert, Bohra Ajay, Bosboom E Marielle H, et al. Effects of wall calcifications in patient-specific wall stress analyses of abdominal aortic aneurysms *Journal of Biomechanical Engineering.* 2007;129:105–109.
15. Li Zhi-Yong, others . Impact of calcification and intraluminal thrombus on the computed wall stresses of abdominal aortic aneurysm *Journal of Vascular Surgery.* 2008;47:928–935.
16. Nagy Róbert, Bojtár Imre. Multimodal biomechanical methods supporting abdominal aortic aneurysm management Biomechanica Hungarica, accepted: 2014 December.
17. Nagy Róbert, Csobay-Novák Csaba, Lovas Attila, Sótonyi Péter, Bojtár Imre. Non-invasive, in vivo strain measurement method in human abdominal aortic aneurysms: Towards a novel approach to rupture risk estimation Journal of Biomechanics, submitted: 2015 January.
18. Hughes Thomas JR, Cottrell John A, Bazilevs Yuri. Isogeometric analysis: CAD, finite elements, NURBS, exact geometry and mesh refinement *Computer methods in applied mechanics and engineering.* 2005;194:4135–4195.
19. Cottrell J.A., Hughes T.J.R., Bazilevs Y.. *Isogeometric Analysis: Toward Integration of CAD and FEA.* Wiley 2009.
20. Holzapfel Gerhard A, Gasser Thomas C, Ogden Ray W. A new constitutive framework for arterial wall mechanics and a comparative study of material models *Journal of elasticity and the physical science of solids.* 2000;61:1–48.

Author: Róbert Nagy
Institute: Department of Structural Mechanics,
Budapest University of Technology and Economics
Street: Műegyetem rkp. 3.
City: Budapest
Country: Hungary
Email: robert.nagy@mail.bme.hu

Modeling of Circular Mass Transport of Nutrients in Capillary Vessels Using Microfluidic Approach

Márton Németh, Ferenc Ender, and András Poppe

Budapest University of Technology and Economics, Department of Electron Devices, Budapest, Hungary

Abstract—

This paper presents a novel reduced order model (ROM), which is applicable to describe the capillary-intercellular space mass-transfer. The model contains the red blood cell (RBC) induced microcirculatory flow. The blood hydrodynamic behavior in capillary vessels can be modeled as a two phase flow, where the phases are the RBC and the plasma. In this flow regime characterized by a low Reynolds number the phases are horizontally alternating and moving along the capillary, so it is similar a the two-phase droplet-flow.

Due to the microcirculation in the two-phase flow higher mass-transfer rates are experienced than in normal laminar flow. In this paper we demonstrate the effect of the microcirculation through the examples of oxygen and LDL transfer, calculated with and without considering the microcirculation in the model. The benefit of using the ROM is the high speed of simulation: by applying our model : the execution time for the same problem is reduced by two orders of magnitude compared to the execution time needed by a detailed CFD model.

Keywords— **capillary vessel, mass-transfer, modeling**

	Nomenclature
c	Concentration (mol/m^3)
$\dot{c}'$	Mass generation rate $(mol/s \cdot m^3)$
$\dot{c}''$	Mass flux $(mol/s \cdot m^2)$
D	Diffusion coefficient (m^2/s)
$\underline{\underline{L_1}}\ \underline{\underline{L_2}}$	First and second part of cylindrical Laplace matrix
l_{plasma}	The simulated length of the plasma phase (m)
P	Capillary wall permeablilty (m^2/s)
r	Radius (m)
Re	Reynolds number
res	Resolution of the model (m)
t	Time (s)
v_{avg}	Average velocity (m/s)
V	Volume (m^3)
$\tau_{circulation}$	Circulation characteristic time (s)
τ_{diff}	Diffusion characteristic time (s)

I. INTRODUCTION

The capillaries are the smallest cross-sectional vessels in the circulatory-system. Their diameters are in the range of 5μm–100μm. The actual mass-transfer between the intravascular and interstitial space takes place in these vessels, therefore the capillary- network is essential for all living tissues. The tissues with higher rate of metabolism require higher density of capillaries, therefore, understanding the capillary mass transfer is very important in cases of certain diseases such as cancer where the ever increasing malignant tumors require more and more nutriments. [1].

Modeling capillaries is among the deeply studied issues in many branches of physiology [2] since with a reliable capillary model the capillary-organ interactions [3] can be better understood. In recent years the approach based on microfluidics has played a major role in such modeling activities, see e.g. [4].

While in the arteries and arterioles we can describe the hydrodynamics of blood-flow with laminar or turbulent flow, in capillaries the flow type is different. The flow characteristics in capillaries can be rather described by a two phase droplet flow. As RBCs are the smallest cells in our organism (with a typical diameter of 6-8μm) they can completely fill the entire cross-section of the smallest capillary vessels resulting in a two-phase flow. Because of the rigidity of RBCs and due the low Reynolds-number a so called droplet flow is formed with the phases of RBC and the plasma. [5]

The droplet-flow is such a special two-phase flow in which the alternating phases are moving in the direction of the flow along the channel. Most frequently CFD (computational fluid dynamics) multi-physics based models are used in a numerical solver to simulate such flows [6]. CFD models are usually accurate but their execution time is impedingly high in medical practice. Therefore our goal is to establish such a model with satisfactory accuracy which can be executed by orders of magnitude faster than a detailed CFD model. The long execution time of CFD calculations is primarily caused by the high mesh density applied during the hydro-dynamical calculations, required especially for the simulation of two phase flows. To eliminate this problem of prohibitively long execution times one may follow two strategies.

One option is the so called *compact modeling* approach can be applied in which a network model is built and solved, following the analogy of the linear differential equations of diffusion (or heat-conduction) and the electrical current. When such a model is created the physical space is divided into small segments and each segment is represented by the circuit equivalent of the corresponding flow section. The newly

Á. Jobbágy (ed.), *First European Biomedical Engineering Conference for Young Investigators*,
IFMBE Proceedings 50, DOI: 10.1007/978-981-287-573-0_25

built circuit can be solved by generally used methods, with constant velocity. The results are close to the CFD-results, and the achievable run-time reduction is around three orders of magnitude [7].
The other way to reduce the long execution time of the detailed CFD models us the so called *reduced order modeling* (ROM). In this approach a behavioral model is created in which calculates the major hydro-dynamical properties without solving the set of the differential equations for all the cells of the detailed CFD mesh. In the following details of such a model representing the two-phase flow in capillary vessels are described.

II. MODELING

Although the analogous problem (heat conduction) was validated with the assistance of detailed CFD simulations and experimental results our novel reduced order model has not been validated yet. The validation of the model can be performed in an alternate way. In the system there is a critical diffusion coefficient, representing a limit between a mostly convectional and a mostly conductional mass transfer. If the reduced order model exhibits a behavior with a similar critical value it can be considered as a proof of correctness of the model.

A. *Governing equations*

The Diffusion-equation is:

$$\frac{\partial c}{\partial t} - D\Delta c = \dot{c}'(\underline{r},t) \tag{1}$$

For cylindrical coordinate system:

$$\frac{\partial c}{\partial t} - \frac{1}{r}\frac{\partial}{\partial r}\left(Dr\frac{\partial c}{\partial r}\right) - \frac{1}{r^2}\frac{\partial}{\partial \phi}D\frac{\partial c}{\partial \phi} - \frac{\partial}{\partial z}D\frac{\partial c}{\partial z} = \dot{c}' \tag{2}$$

By applying the finite difference method we get the following matrix equation for the concentration in the mesh nodes:

$$\underline{\underline{c}}(\underline{r},t+dt) = \underline{\underline{r,}}\,\underline{c}(t) + \frac{dt}{res^2}\underline{\underline{\alpha}}\left(\underline{\underline{L_1}}\cdot\underline{\underline{c}}(\underline{r},t) + \underline{\underline{c}}(\underline{r},t)\cdot\underline{\underline{L_2}}^{\dagger}\right), \tag{3}$$

where *res* is the spatial resolution finite difference of the reduced order model. WThe $\underline{\underline{L_1}}$ and $\underline{\underline{L_2}}$ matrices to represent the Laplace operator for cylindrical coordinate system. The matrices used in Eq. (**??**) look as follows:

$$\underline{\underline{\alpha}}_{i,j} = D_{i,j}, \tag{4}$$

where $D_{i,j}$ is filled by the diffusion coefficient of material in the mesh cell i, j. The $\underline{\underline{L}}$ matrices are:

$$\underline{\underline{L_1}}_{i,j} = -2\delta_{i,j} + \delta_{i+1,j} + \delta_{i,j+1} \tag{5}$$

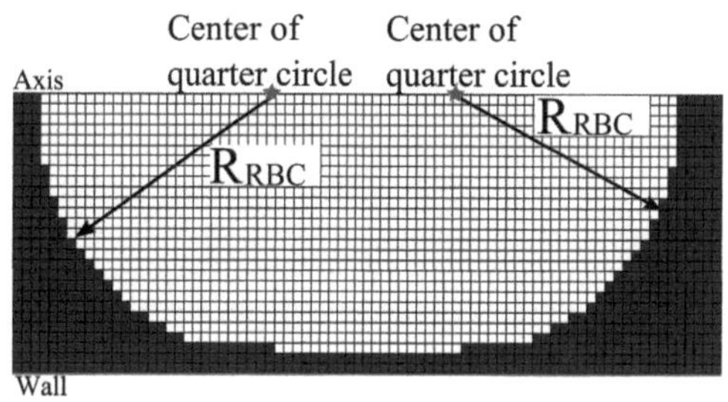

Fig. 1: The phase boundaries in the simulation mesh: the white area represents an RBC, the dark blue area represents the plasma.

$$\underline{\underline{L_2}}_{i,j} = -2\delta_{i,j} + \left(1 - \frac{1}{2(j-0.5)}\right)\delta_{i,j+1} + \left(1 + \frac{1}{2(j-0.5)}\right)\delta_{i+1,j} \tag{6}$$

where j is the radial coordinate. $j-0.5$ is the middle radius between two neighboring nodes.

B. *Initialization*

The modeled capillary blood vessel section has a length of 1 mm and its radius is 5.4 μm. We choose a 0.2-by-0.2 μm equidistant square-mesh which resulted in 135000 nodes. The simulated physical time of the flow was 1.5s. The RBC boundaries were fixed (pre-defined) in the reduced order model, see Figure 1. The phase lengths are 60μm for the plasma, and 30μm for the blood cells phase. The considered length of RBCs was much longer than the thickness of the free RBCs because the red blood cells are deformed in the capillary. [8]

C. *Boundary conditions*

Boundary conditions are imposed at the edges of the simulated zone and at the phase boundaries.
At the *Inlet* an alternating phase boundary is assumed with constant velocity.
The *outlet* is a simple outflow, without any consideration.
At the *wall* Neumann-boundary condition is applied with $\dot{c}''(\underline{r},t) = P\cdot(c_{wall} - c_{interstitial})$ flux, where P is the permeability of the capillary wall.
To apply these boundary conditions the $\underline{\underline{L}}$ matrices need to be modified in first an last rows (columns). Which was done before implementation.

D. *Microcirculation*

The specialty of the droplet flow is the high rate of the radial heat and mass transport which is due to the so called

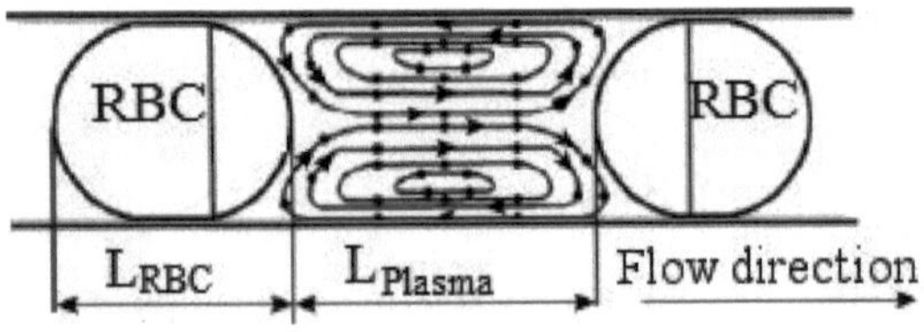

Fig. 2: Circulation in droplet [9]

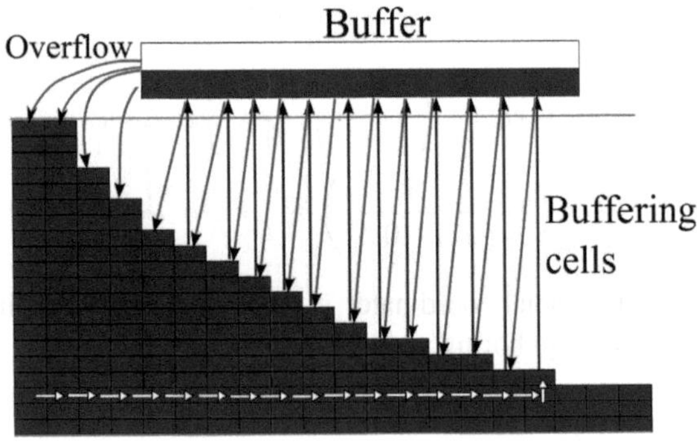

Fig. 3: The method of circulation implementation

microcirculation as illustrated in Figure 2. The circulation realizes a transport path between the wall and the center of the droplet. If the flow trajectories are known then the only difficulty in modeling the microcirculation in axisymmetric geometries is that the simulation segment volumes corresponding to the different radii are also different. This problem can be solved by the introduction of a *buffer* for the simulation of movement of the segments. With this buffer the steps of modeling the movement of the segments are as follows. First, the buffer is filled with material in the volume of the actual segment and the concentration of the buffer is also set to the segment concentration. Then we reduce the volume of the buffer by the volume of the new, subsequent segment and the concentration of this subsequent segment is set equal to the concentration of the buffer. This is repeated until the residual volume is bigger than the volume of the subsequent segment. In case of a new segment entered into the flow the buffer volume is set to the sum the volume of the new segment and the residual volume and the buffer concentration will be the concentration calculated for the mixture of the two volumes. This process can be followed in Figure 3. As we get closer to the axis of the capillary the segment volumes get smaller, therefore the flow velocity must be increased to satisfy continuity. The circulation model can also be applied to the inner layers of the segments of the flow model.

E. Modeling the mass transfer

The mass transfer, i.e. the movement of the phase-boundaries is modeled as follows. We assume a dt time step for which the Courant–Friedrichs–Lewy (CFL) condition is satisfied:

$$dt \leq 0.5\frac{res^2}{D} \tag{7}$$

With this simulation time step the time evolution of the concentration is calculated according to the relation $c(t+dt) = c(t) + dt \cdot L_1 \ldots$ obtained from the diffusion-equation. At every time-step the concentration of the phase-boundary and the new concentration is calculated. After a simulation time increment reaches the $t = res/v$ time, the model is advanced by one mesh grid cell in the direction of the flow – affecting the phase boundaries and the concentration distribution. At the same time we determine for every segment of the released one mesh grid-cell wide region at the inlet side of the simulation domain the phase (RBC or plasma). Then calculations for the circulation take place at the same time.

The effect of the microcirculation is dominant, if the circulation time is similar or less than the diffusion characteristic time.

According to [7] the circulation time is approximately

$$\tau_{circulation} = \frac{l_{plasma}}{v_{avg}} = 0.03s, \tag{8}$$

with $v_{avg} = 2mm/s$. The characteristic time for diffusion is:

$$\tau_{diff} = \frac{r^2}{D} = \frac{2.92 \cdot 10^{-11}}{D} s \tag{9}$$

In this regime, the critical diffusion coefficient:

$$\tau_{circulation} = \tau_{diff} \Rightarrow D_{crit} \simeq 9.72 \cdot 10^{-10} \sim 10^{-9} m^2/s. \tag{10}$$

III. RESULTS

The model was implemented in Matlab 2013a. The initial concentrations were $0.0005 mol/m^3$ for each substrate, the wall permeability was set to $P = 0.00015 m^2/s$, the average velocity was assumed to be $v_{avg} = 2mm/s$. For each simulation the parameters were identical except the diffusion coefficients of the substrates which were set to $D_{trial} = 10^{-8} m^2/s$, $D_O = 10^{-9} m^2/s$, and $D_{LDL} = 10^{-11} m^2/s$ as a trial, for oxygen, and for the LDL cholesterol respectively. The results are shown in Figure 4. where the radial dependence of the concentration is shown at the same 218μm axial position.The results for the the cases when the diffusion coefficient exceeds the D_{crit} critical diffusion coefficient (1st case), when it is close the D_{crit} ($2^{nd} case$) and when it is below D_{crit} (3rd

case) are well distinguishable. For the 1st case there is no significant difference between the micro-circulational and non-circulational curves. In the 3rd case the difference is very conspicuous: the curves are very dissimilar. The effect of the microcirculation in the 2nd case is visible it is considerable. In this case the conductive and convective mass transfer is almost identical, resulting in an almost stagnating circulational curve.

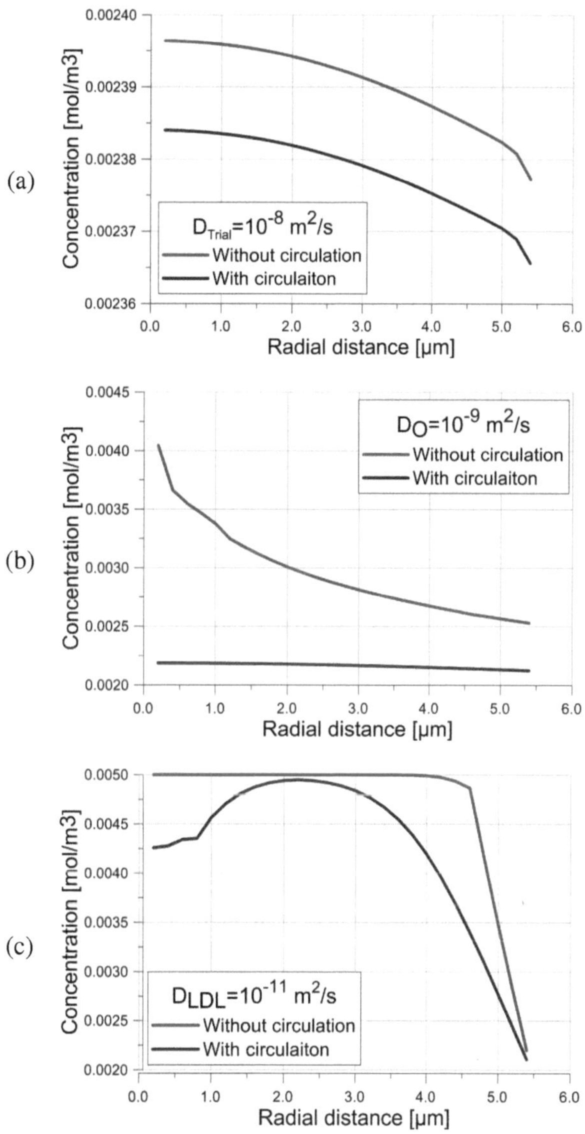

Fig. 4: The concentration dependence on the radius, with (red), and without (blue) the microcirculations for three cases of the concentration: (a) $D = 10^{-8}m^2/s$, (b) $D = 10^{-9}m^2/s$, (c) $D = 10^{-11}m^2/s$ cases

IV. Conclusions

A reduced order model for the description of mass transfer in capillary vessels was proposed. As a first test of the model the critical behavior was simulated. The obtained results meet the theoretical expectations suggesting that this model can be well applied as a behavioral model of the capillary blood flow. As a next step, a detailed A CFD model of this flow will be created to allow a precise validation of our reduced order model.

With the present model we found that the microcirculation caused by the RBCs results in higher mass transfer rates. This has to be taken into consideration when the diffusion coefficient is below the (velocity and radius dependent) critical diffusion coefficient of the substrates.

References

1. Gazit Yuval, Berk David A, Leunig Michael, Baxter Laurence T, Jain Rakesh K. Scale-invariant behavior and vascular network formation in normal and tumor tissue *Physical review letters.* 1995;75:2428.
2. Spiess Bruce D. Perfluorocarbon emulsions as a promising technology: a review of tissue and vascular gas dynamics *Journal of Applied Physiology.* 2009;106:1444–1452.
3. Sourbron SP, Buckley DL. Tracer kinetic modelling in MRI: estimating perfusion and capillary permeability *Physics in medicine and biology.* 2012;57:R1.
4. Wong Keith HK, Chan Juliana M, Kamm Roger D, Tien Joe. Microfluidic models of vascular functions *Annual review of biomedical engineering.* 2012;14:205–230.
5. Prothero J, Burton AC. The physics of blood flow in capillaries: I. The nature of the motion *Biophysical journal.* 1961;1:565.
6. Gupta Raghvendra, Fletcher David F, Haynes Brian S. On the CFD modelling of Taylor flow in microchannels *Chemical Engineering Science.* 2009;64:2941–2950.
7. Ender Ferenc, Németh Márton, Pálovics Péter, Drozdy Andras, Poppe András. Thermal compact modeling approach of droplet microreactor based Lab-on-a-Chip devices *Microelectronics Journal.* 2014;45:1786–1794.
8. Jeong Jae Hong, Sugii Yasusiko, Minamiyama Motomu, Okamoto Koji. Measurement of RBC deformation and velocity in capillaries in vivo *Microvascular research.* 2006;71:212–217.
9. CAI Wangfeng, ZHANG Jiao, ZHANG Xubin, WANG Yan, QI Xiangjuan. Enhancement of CO_2 Absorption under Taylor Flow in the Presence of Fine Particles *Chinese Journal of Chemical Engineering.* 2013;21:135–143.

Corresponding author: Márton Németh, Budapest University of Technology and Economics, Department of Electron Devices, Budapest, 1117 Magyar tudósok körútja 2., Q, 3. floor, Hungary. E-mail: nemeth@eet.bme.hu

Reduced Order Thermal Modeling of Gas-Liquid Droplet-Flow

Márton Németh and András Poppe

Budapest University of Technology and Economics, Department of Electron Devices, Budapest, Hungary

Abstract— **The paper presents a reduced order thermal model, which enables the thermal analysis of two-phase Taylor-flow. Two-phase Taylor flow is the basis of many microfluidic applications such as bio-chemical microreactors where segmented zones are required to accurately characterize enzyme reactions. This new model represents a microtube with horizontally alternating and moving liquid and gas phases. The results obtained by the reduced order model match the results of a validated detailed Ansys-Fluent model with 5% accuracy. The reduced order model accounts for microcirculation and back flow. The proposed reduced order model of the two-phase Taylor-flow is investigated in situations characterized by different Reynolds numbers.**

Keywords— **Compact thermal modeling, segmented slug flow, Lab-on-a-Chip, calorimetry**

	Nomenclature
A_{Bubble}	Cross-sectional area of the bubble $[m^2]$
c_V	Volumetric specific heat capacity $[J/m^3K]$
δ_F	Fluid film thickness $[m]$
λ	Thermal conductivity $[W/m \cdot K]$
$\underline{\underline{L_1}}\ \underline{\underline{L_2}}$	First and second part of the cylindrical Laplace matrix
$\dot{q}'$	Heat generation rate $[W/m^3]$
$\dot{q}''$	Heat flux $[W/m^2]$
r	Radius $[m]$
Re	Reynolds number
res	Resolution of the model $[m]$
ρ	Density $[kg/m^3]$
T	Temperature $[K]$
ΔT_{Avg}	Average temperature rise on wall $[K]$
t	Time $[s]$
v	Average velocity $[m/s]$
V	Volume $[m^3]$

I. INTRODUCTION

The growing interest in Lab-on-Chip (LoC) platforms requires fast and accurate models to describe the thermal behavior of microchannels. While the complexity of the devices is growing, the attempts to create fast and accurate reduced order models of such devices have not been completely successful yet.

Bio-chemical microreactors are among the most important applications of microfluidics. The achievable reduction of sample volume and the expected high throughput are the motivations to design and manufacture microreactors. . Chemical microreactors are often completed with microcalorimetry, which is a non-labeled sensing method for almost every chemical reaction. It is based on the heat generation of the reaction. During a bio-chemical reaction the heat generation density is low as a consequence of the low concentrations of the reagents. The consequence of the low heat generation density accompanied by the small volume is that microcalorimetry requires to measure very small temperature differences caused by the reaction heat [1]. This means that accurate and very sensitive thermometers equipped with signal processing circuitry need to be integrated into the microreactors. The focus of this paper is the design of such systems by the application of a reduced order thermal model of the microchannel with the flow of reagents, which is a so called two-phase Taylor-flow.

Due to the low heat generation, proper description (modeling) of the channel-channel interactions is important in the design process. The ultimate goal of the paper is to open a new path in modeling to support the design of complex microfluidic systems, by taking into account the interaction between the microchannels.

II. MODELING

Our new reduced order model was validated with the help of detailed CFD simulations with parameter settings described in [2]. Our present work is based on the paper of Gupta et al [3]. Since their CFD simulation results were validated by actual experiments [4] and the CFD accuracy was also investigated by Aland et al [5], we considered the detailed CFD model based multi-physical simulation experiments as a reliable reference, equivalent to real physical experiments. Using data obtained from these simulation experiments we could estimate the errors of our reduced order model.

A. Governing equations

The Fourier-equation of heat conduction:

$$c_V \frac{\partial T}{\partial t} - \lambda \Delta T = \dot{q}'(\underline{r},t) \tag{1}$$

Á. Jobbágy (ed.), *First European Biomedical Engineering Conference for Young Investigators*,
IFMBE Proceedings 50, DOI: 10.1007/978-981-287-573-0_26

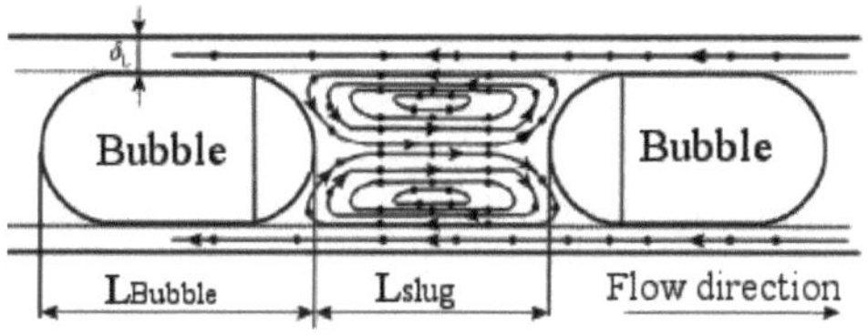

Figure 1: Fluid circulation in a droplet [6]

which for cylindrical coordinate system is:

$$c_V \frac{\partial T}{\partial t} - \frac{1}{r}\frac{\partial}{\partial r}\left(\lambda r \frac{\partial T}{\partial r}\right) - \frac{1}{r^2}\frac{\partial}{\partial \phi}\lambda\frac{\partial T}{\partial \phi} - \frac{\partial}{\partial z}\lambda\frac{\partial T}{\partial z} = \dot{q}' \quad (2)$$

Discretizing it for the numerical solution we get a formula describing the time evolution of heat propagation:

$$\underline{\underline{T}}(t+dt) = \underline{\underline{T}}(t) + \frac{dt}{res^2}\underline{\underline{\alpha}}\left(\underline{\underline{L_1}} \cdot \underline{\underline{T}}(t) + \underline{\underline{T}}(t) \cdot \underline{\underline{L_2}}^{\dagger}\right) \quad (3)$$

where *res* is the spatial resolution of the reduced order model (constant both for the radial and axial directions). The $\underline{\underline{L_1}}$ and $\underline{\underline{L_2}}$ matrices represent the Laplace operator for cylindrical coordinate system. The matrices used in Eq. (3) look as follows:

$$\underline{\underline{\alpha}}_{i,j} = \frac{\lambda_{i,j}}{c_{i,j}} \quad (4)$$

$$\underline{\underline{L_1}}_{i,j} = -2\delta_{i,j} + \delta_{i+1,j} + \delta_{i,j+1} \quad (5)$$

$$\underline{\underline{L_2}}_{i,j} = -2\delta_{i,j} + \left(1 - \frac{1}{2(j-0.5)}\right)\delta_{i,j+1} + \left(1 + \frac{1}{2(j-0.5)}\right)\delta_{i+1,j} \quad (6)$$

where j is the radial coordinate (in multiples of *res*). The value $j-0.5$ is the length of the middle radius between adjacent nodes.

B. Microcirculation and backflow

The specialty of the droplet flow is the high radial heat and mass transport which is due to the so called *microcirculation* as illustrated in Figure 1. The circulation realizes a transport path between the wall and the center of the droplet. For the sake of accurate modeling the heat transfer realized by the microcirculation also needs to be accounted for during the simulation. If the flow trajectories are known the only difficulty in modeling the microcirculation in axisymmetric geometries is that the simulation cell volumes corresponding to the different radii are also different. This problem can be solved by the introduction of a *buffering storage object* or *buffer* for the simulation of movement of the cells. With this buffer the steps of modeling the movement of the cells are as follows. First the buffer is filled with material in the volume of the actual cell and the temperature of the buffer is also set to the cell temperature. Then we reduce the volume of the buffer by the volume of the new, subsequent cell and the temperature of this subsequent cell is set equal to the temperature of the buffer. This is repeated until the residual volume is bigger than the volume of the subsequent cell. In case of a new cell entered into the flow the buffer volume is set to the sum the volume of the new cell and the residual volume and the buffer temperature will be the temperature calculated for the mixture of the two volumes. This process can be followed in Figure 2. As we get closer to the axis of the microchannel the cell volumes get smaller, therefore the flow velocity must increase to satisfy continuity. The circulation model can also be applied to inner layers of cells of the flow model. According to the *Armand-relation* the speed of the movement of the gas phase is higher than the speed of the fluid. This results in a back-flow in the system. According to experimental data the ratio of the velocity of the gas phase and the average speed is 1.2. In an accurate model both the Armand-relation and the back-flow must be taken into account. The speed of the back-flow can be determined from the differences of the (volumetric) flow velocities. As the back-flow takes place around the bubbles (at their boundaries), the velocity of the back-flow can be determined from the cross-sectional area of the bubbles. The volumes of fluid entering a droplet and the corresponding flow velocities also need to be handled properly. For solving this issue our assumption is that the velocity of the back-flow is uniform in all simulation grid cells along the channel walls.

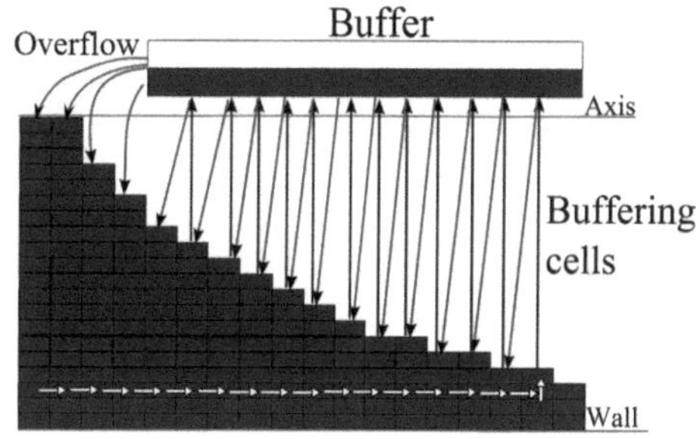

Figure 2: The method of implementation of modeling the microcirculation

C. Initialization

The modeled channel has a 3 mm length and its radius is 162 μm. We choose a 6-by-6 μm equidistant square-mesh which resulted in 13500 nodes. The phase boundaries were

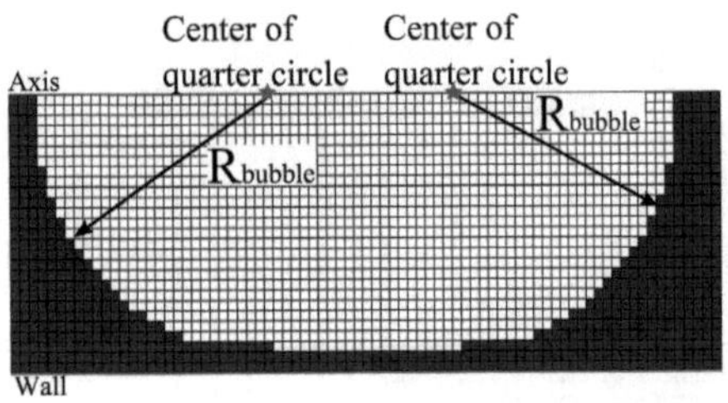

Figure 3: The phase boundaries (a bubble) in the simulation mesh.

fixed (pre-defined) in the reduced order model, see Figure 3. The heat generation is adjusted to a Neumann boundary condition with $\dot{q}'' = 100W/m^2$ along the wall.

D. Modeling the mass transfer

The mass transfer, i.e. the movement of the phase-boundaries is modeled as follows. We assume a dt time step for which the Courant–Friedrichs–Lewy (CFL) condition is satisfied, so $dt \leq 0.5\frac{\lambda res}{cv}$. With this simulation time step the time evolution of the temperature field is calculated according to the relation $T(t+dt) = T(t) + dt \cdot L_1 \ldots$ obtained from the Fourier-law of heat conduction. As the simulation time is advanced, different events may take place in the model. At every time-step the temperature of the phase-boundary and the new temperature field has to be calculated. After $t_{n,1}$ of time, the whole system is advanced by one grid cell in the direction of the flow. At the same time we determine for every cell of the released one grid-cell wide region at the inlet side of the simulation domain what is the type of the phase (gas or fluid). Then the back-flow is simulated at $t_{n,2}$: the grid cells which are between the channel wall and the phase boundary are moved by one position backwards (towards the inlet, in the opposite direction of the main flow). The major steps of the simulation can be summarized as follows:

1. Satisfy the boundary conditions (phase boundary): the temperature at the phase boundary is re-calculated
2. Solve equation (3) to advance the model in time by dt
3. The entire contents of the channel is advanced in space by a single grid-cell in the direction of the flow ($t_{flow} = t_{n,1}$)
4. At the inlet side of the simulation domain the released cells are filled with the right phase (bubble or fluid) material ($t_{flow} = t_{n,1}$)
5. Move backwards the contents of the cells, which are affected by the back-flow ($t_{flow} = t_{n,2}$)
6. Calculate the microcirculation ($t_{flow} = t_{n,2}$)

Steps 3 and 4 are executed only if the simulation time reached one of the $t_{n,1} = 1.2\frac{n \cdot l}{v}$ instances (where $l = 6\mu$m, and n is a positive integer), i.e. if the distance travelled by the gas phase is already equal to the size of a grid cell.

Steps 5 and 6 are executed if the velocity of the back-flow necessitates these calculations, i.e. the grid cells in the back-flow region are moved backwards by one position when the distance calculated from the black-flow velocity is equal to the cell width. This velocity can be calculated as follows:

$$v_{Backflow} = \frac{\Delta v_{phase} A_{bub}}{A_{out-bub}} = 0.2\frac{r_{bub}^2}{(r_{chan} - res)^2 - r_{bub}^2}, \quad (7)$$

where A_{bub}, $A_{out-bub}$, r_{chan} are the bubble phase maximal cross-sectional area, the outside cross-sectional area of the bubble ($\pi r_{chan}^2 - A_{Bub}$)and the channel radius, respectively. Δv is the velocity difference between the phases, as given by the Armand-relation. So steps 5 and 6 are executed only if the simulation time reaches one of the $t_{n,2} = \frac{n \cdot res}{v_{Backflow}}$ instances.

III. Results for different Reynolds numbers

The results obtained for different Reynolds numbers are shown in Figure 4. The most problematic region is at the front of the profile since in the Ansys-Fluent model the calculation of the bubble shaping process is included, while in our reduced order model we calculate with a fixed shape, pre-defined phase boundary at the bubbles.

The accuracy of the compact model was investigated at different flow rates. The axial temperature distribution was calculated in the slug sections both in Ansys-Fluent and by solving the reduced order model. The resulted functions were compared and the *variance* (σ^2) of the two temperature profiles was calculated as follows:

$$\sigma^2 = \frac{1}{N}\sum_{i=1}^{N}(T_{\mathrm{FLT}}(x_i) - T_{\mathrm{ROM}}(x_i))^2, \quad (8)$$

where N is the number of nodes to sum. To calculate the relative error the variance was compared to the average temperature rise:

$$Err_\sigma = \frac{\sigma^2}{\sum_{i=1}^{500}(\Delta T_{\mathrm{FLT}}(x_i)/500)} \quad (9)$$

The errors are detailed in Table 1. The relative error is around 5%, therefore our novel reduced order model is suitable for the description of thermally coupled microfluidic systems.

IV. Conclusion

Based on the general properties of the segmented flow, such as microcirculation and back-flow, a reduced order

Re	σ^2 of temperature profile (K^2)	Average temperature rise (K)	Relative error(%)
1	$4.86 \cdot 10^{-5}$	0.158	4.41
3	$9.06 \cdot 10^{-6}$	0.067	4.49
5	$6.45 \cdot 10^{-6}$	0.051	4.98
7	$5.35 \cdot 10^{-6}$	0.043	5.38

Table 1: Model accuracy for different flow rates under constant heat flux at the wall

model is proposed to describe heat transfer in microchannels. Thermal analysis was performed by this novel reduced order model which was validated by comparisons to the results of a detailed CFD model used in Ansys-Fluent. The reduced order model is at least by two orders of magnitude faster than the detailed CFD model solved by Ansys-Fluent. The difference between the temperature profiles calculated by the two models is around 5% for a wide range of Reynolds-numbers. Considering the reduced simulation times and the accuracy, our proposed reduced order model can be effectively used in the design of complex microfluidic systems. The model is suitable to improve the description of thermally-coupled microchannel systems.

REFERENCES

1. Lee Wonhee, Fon Warren, Axelrod Blake W, Roukes Michael L. High-sensitivity microfluidic calorimeters for biological and chemical applications *Proceedings of the National Academy of Sciences.* 2009;106:15225–15230.
2. Ender Ferenc, Németh Márton, Pálovics Péter, Drozdy Andras, Poppe András. Thermal compact modeling approach of droplet microreactor based Lab-on-a-Chip devices *Microelectronics Journal.* 2014.
3. Gupta Raghvendra, Fletcher David F., Haynes Brian S.. CFD modelling of flow and heat transfer in the Taylor flow regime *Chemical Engineering Science.* 2010;65:2094–2107.
4. Asadolahi Azadeh N., Gupta Raghvendra, Leung Sharon S.Y., Fletcher David F., Haynes Brian S.. Validation of a CFD model of Taylor flow hydrodynamics and heat transfer *Chemical Engineering Science.* 2012;69:541–552.
5. Aland Sebastian, Lehrenfeld Christoph, Marschall Holger, Meyer Christoph, Weller Stephan. Accuracy of two-phase flow simulations: The Taylor Flow benchmark *PAMM.* 2013;13:595–598.
6. CAI Wangfeng, ZHANG Jiao, ZHANG Xubin, WANG Yan, QI Xiangjuan. Enhancement of CO_2 Absorption under Taylor Flow in the Presence of Fine Particles *Chinese Journal of Chemical Engineering.* 2013;21:135–143.

Corresponding author: Márton Németh, Budapest University of Technology and Economics, Department of Electron Devices, Budapest, 1117 Magyar tudósok körútja 2., Q, 3. floor, Hungary. E-mail: nemeth@eet.bme.hu

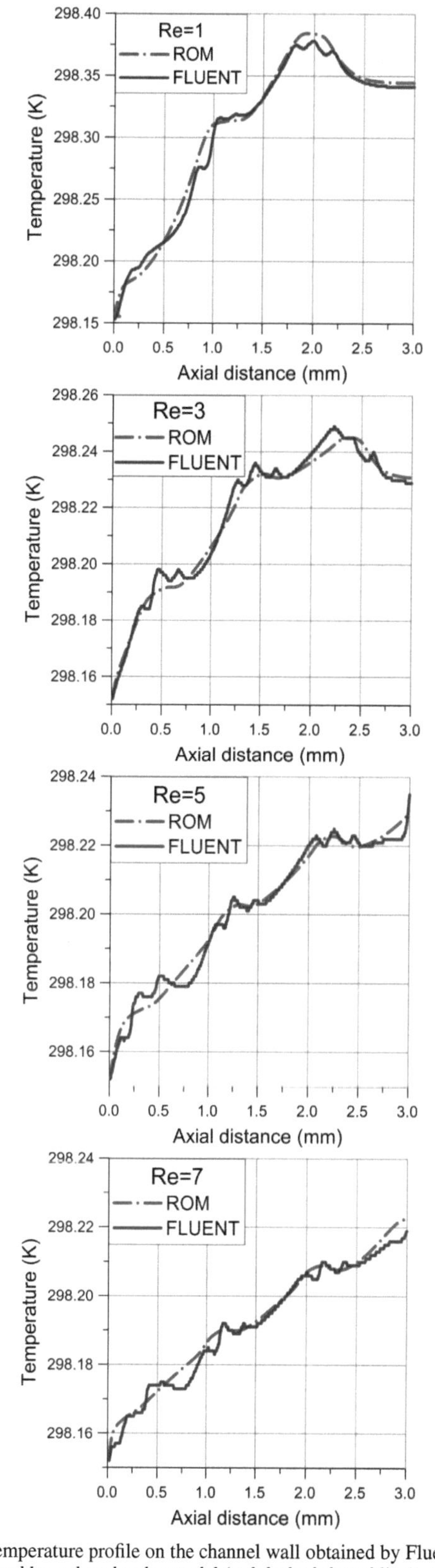

Figure 4: Temperature profile on the channel wall obtained by Fluent (blue, solid line) and by reduced order model (red dashed-dotted line), $Re = 1$–7

Association of Autoantibody Levels with the Hazard of Autoimmune Comorbidities in Children with Type 1 Diabetes

T. Ferenci[1], A. Körner[2], and L. Kovács[1]

[1] Óbuda University, John von Neumann Faculty of Informatics, Physiological Controls Group, Budapest, Hungary
[2] Semmelweis University, 1st Department of Paediatrics, Budapest, Hungary

Abstract— **Type 1 diabetes mellitus is an autoimmune disease representing serious burden both on the patients and healthcare systems. Being an autoimmune disease it comes as no surprise that it is often associated with other autoimmune comorbidities, such as coeliac disease or Hashimoto's thyroiditis. As the manifestation of these diseases is often preceded by a longer period of latent (subclinical) autoimmune process, children diagnosed with type 1 diabetes mellitus are often screened for autoantibodies characteristic for these comorbidities to predict their occurrence. Data from $n = 182$ children diagnosed with type 1 diabetes mellitus undergoing such screening program were collected from 2007 to 2012. Cox proportional hazards model with time varying covariate was used to model how autoantibody levels are associated with the hazard of the onset of an autoimmune comorbidity. For coeliac disease, only the IgA subclass of anti-transglutaminase autoantibodies turned out to be relevant ($p < 0.0001$), with a hazard ratio – for being >10 U/ml compared to being smaller – of 44.8 (95% HR: 11.88-168.8). For Hashimoto's thyroiditis, only anti-thyroid peroxidase autoantibodies were significant ($p < 0.0001$), with a hazard ratio raising rapidly to roughly 10 by 100 U/ml, then – after a sharp break in the gradient – raising much more slowly to about 30-40 for the extreme ATPO values greater than 1000 U/ml. This study confirmed the role of autoantibodies in predicting autoimmune comorbidities in T1DM and also demonstrated a way to quantify this effect.**

Keywords— **Type 1 diabetes mellitus, autoimmunity, autoantibody, comorbidities, proportional hazards model with time varying covariates.**

I. INTRODUCTION

Type 1 of diabetes mellitus (T1DM) is a prototypical example of autoimmune diseases, in which a T_H1-mediated autoimmune process destroys the insulin-producing β-cells in the pancreatic islets [1]. The resulting absolute or almost absolute deficiency in insulin hinders the entry of glucose from blood to glucose-consuming cells leading to short-term and long-term complications and consequences, even in the presence of adequate treatment [2].

It is very old observation that those patients who have an autoimmune disease (AID) are prone to have a second (or further) AID. In addition to anecdotal evidence, corroborating lessons learned from animal experiments [3] and results of genome-wide association analysis [4, 5], this statement is now supported by epidemiological studies as well, although often of varying quality [6, 7]. Also, it is largely unclear whether this is a general risk among AIDs, or there are certain combinations that emerge more frequently. Nevertheless, it is accepted that in T1DM, the risk of coeliac disease and Hashimoto's thyroiditis is substantially increased [8]; these will be in focus of the present study.

Coeliac disease (CD) is an AID characterized by an abnormal inflammatory response to the dietary exposure to gliadian (a protein found in wheat) and related gluten proteins, which leads to villous atrophy in the small intestine, leading to malabsorption symptoms, among others [9]. Occurrence of CD is strongly associated with T1DM [10] that the screening for the signs of CD, most notably elevated autoantibody-levels is often recommended [11].

Hashimoto's thyroiditis (HT) is an autoimmune thyroiditis, characterized by the lymphocytic invasion of the thyroid tissue, the destruction of which will give rise to hypothyroidism [12]. HT is also strongly associated with T1DM [13, 14].

It is now recognized that the onset of most AIDs is not an abrupt event, rather, a result of a longer process, most of which is subclinical [15]. This gives rise to the possibility to predict the disease before its manifestation. A prime example for such approaches is the screening [16] for autoantibodies: the presence of autoantibodies is not the same as the presence of manifest disease, however they can be used if the presumption is accepted that their level is already elevated in the latent period of the autoimmune process [17].

The present paper will investigate the relationship between autoantibody levels characteristic for CD and HT and the manifestion of these diseases among children suffering in T1DM.

Á. Jobbágy (ed.), *First European Biomedical Engineering Conference for Young Investigators*,
IFMBE Proceedings 50, DOI: 10.1007/978-981-287-573-0_27

II. MATERIALS AND METHODS

A. Patient data

$n = 182$ children suffering in T1DM were selected as a convenience sample from patients treated at the 1st Department of Paediatrics of the Semmelweis University. Autoantibodies that are characteristic for CD and HT were measured annually from 2007 (or from the inclusion in the study, i.e. onset of DM) to 2012. Only those subjects were included in the present study who had no clinically manifest CD or HT at the manifestation of the DM, as the "index disease" was DM in the present study. In addition to basic sociodemographic data (sex, date of birth) and the date of DM onset, the onset of clinically manifest CD and HT – if there was – was also recorded. Patient characteristics are summarized in Table 1.

Table 1: Characteristics of the patients included in the study. Categorical variables are presented as frequencies and percentages, continuous variables are presented in Mean (Median) ± SD (IQR) [Min-Max] format.

Parameter	Descriptive statistics
Sex	96 male (52.7%), 86 female (47.3%)
Age at the onset of DM	7.7 (8.0) ± 4.3 (7.0) [0-17]
Distribution of manifest autoimmune comorbidities	None: 142 (78.0%), only CD: 22 (12.1%), only HT: 12 (6.6%), both CD and HT: 6 (3.3%)
Time to CD onset (from DM onset) for CD cases	3.0 (1.0) ± 2.3 (2.2) [1-10]
Time to HT onset (from DM onset) for HT cases	5.4 (5.0) ± 3.0 (4.8) [1-11]

The measured autoantibodies were:

- Anti-transglutaminase, both IgA and IgG subclasses (TGIgA, TGIgG). These autoantibodies are characteristic for CD as tissue transglutaminase (tTG) is recognized as the autoantigene in the disease [18]: tTG has a role in the post-translational modification of certain wheat gluten proteins; antibodies directed against them play role in the villous destruction [19, 20].
- Anti-thyroid peroxidase (ATPO) and anti-thyroglobulin (ATG). These thyroid autoantibodies are present in the majority of the HT cases [21].

TGIgA and TGIgG were binarized at 10 U/ml, which was just the upper bound of the reference range, as the vast majority of the measurements were having a value of exactly 5, thus there was no point in handling these as continuous variables.

ATPO and ATG were logarithmized to account for their heavily skewed distribution. Scatter plot between the two is show on Figure 1. Note that this scatter plot shows every measurement equally, regardless of the subject and year of measurement, i.e. it neglects the possible intra-individual correlations.

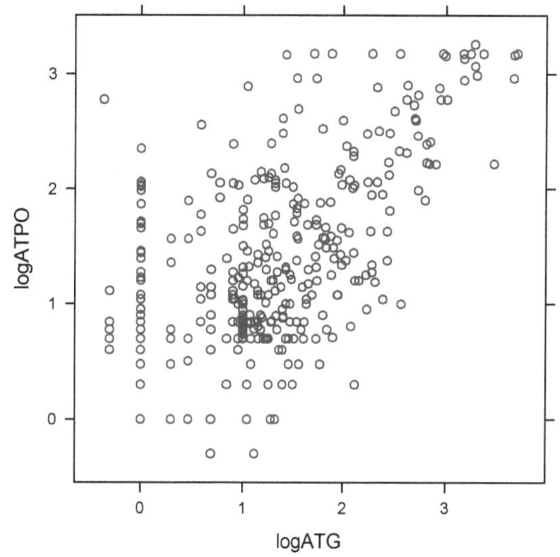

Fig. 1: Scatter plot of logATG and logATPO across the whole sample.

B. Statistical analysis

The collected data can be considered to be time-to-event data, where time is measured from the onset of T1DM, and the – non-recurring – event is the onset of clinically manifest CD or HT. (These two will be considered in two separate analysis.) Thus, the apparatus of survival analysis [22] can be applied, in particular, Cox proportional hazards model [23] will be used, as it casts the problem in regression framework, making it possible to study the effects of certain covariates on survival. These covariates are considered to be multiplicatively affecting the so-called baseline hazard; thus the term "proportional hazards" model. Proportionality will be assessed with the test of Grambsch and Therneua [24]. The achieve our stated aim, the covariates will be the measured autoantibody levels. Sex and age at the onset of T1DM will also be added to the model, to control for their possible confounding effect. For continuous variables, flexibility in functional form specification will be achieved by using spline regression with restricted cubic splines [25]. After model diagnostics and model selection (with LR-test for nested models), the final model will be validated in terms of discrimination using bootstrap [26].

In this setting, autoantibody levels are classical examples of time varying (time dependent) covariates, as their value changes from year to year. Thus, appropriate model has to be applied to incorporate such covariates [23, 27].

To perform the calculations, version 3.1.1 of the `R` program package [28] together with the `survival` [29] and `rms` [30] libraries was applied, using a custom script developed for this purpose which is available at the corresponding author on request.

III. RESULTS

A. Coeliac disease

The interaction between the subclasses of anti-transglutaminase autoantibodies, and sex and age at DM onset are irrelevant ($p = 0.9758$). Interestingly, IgG is also irrelevant in the obtained model ($p = 0.1186$), and also with the aforementioned covariates ($p = 0.4979$), leaving IgA subclass of anti-transglutaminase autoantibody the only covariate, which is however relevant ($p < 0.0001$).

The obtained model passes the proportionality test ($p = 0.699$), and has an R^2 of 43.7%, which is still 41.8% with bootsrap validation.

In this final model the coefficient of anti-transglutaminase IgA is 3.8, giving rise to a hazard ratio of 44.8 (if the autoantibody level is above 10 U/ml), with a 95% confidence interval of 11.88-168.8.

B. Hashimoto's thyroiditis

Sex and age at DM onset, and nonlinearities in ATG were irrelevant even together ($p = 0.4726$). Even after leaving out these covariates, ATG itself is still irrelevant ($p = 0.1173$, and $p = 0.2639$ together), so the final model only includes ATPO (but with splines).

This model passes proportionality test ($p = 0.731$) and has an R^2 of 29.5%, which is 26.3% under bootstrap validation.

Overall, ATPO is relevant at $p < 0.001$; with hazard ratio given on Figure 2.

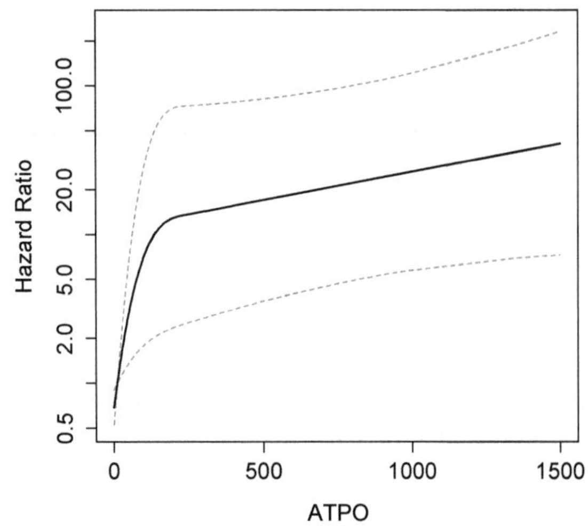

Fig. 2: Hazard ratio for different levels of ATPO, estimated with restricted cubic spline.

IV. DISCUSSION AND CONCLUSION

Interestingly IgG subclass of anti-transglutaminase autoantibodies did not turn out to be a relevant factor in explaining the hazard of CD in children with T1DM. While it might be due to the relatively low sample size, it also worth mentioning that several other studies also found that IgG is less reliable for CD [31]. In contrast, IgA had a hazard ratio in excess to 40 (if it is above 10 U/ml, compared to being smaller than this threshold).

As far as HT is concerned, only ATPO turned out to be relevant. This had a nonlinear impact on hazard ratio: until about 100 U/ml (note that the upper bound of the reference range is 35 with the exception of the first year, when it was 63) it raises rapidly to roughly 10, then there is a sharp break in the gradient, and raises much more slowly to about 30-40 for the extreme ATPO values greater than 1000 U/ml. It is important to mention that at this range, the confidence interval is very large (even for 1500 U/ml, it spans from 5 to 200) due to the very small number of observations with such extreme ATPO values.

Naturally, our study also has certain limitations. The first and foremost – in addition to the convenience sampling – is perhaps the fact that subjects were followed only from 2007, irrespectively of the onset of their DM. It would have given a more accurate picture, if subjects were all followed right since the onset of their DM.

Another limitation is the fact that the values of antibody levels were considered themselves, without regard to the previous/further measurements within the same subject. In other words, the possible effect of certain time-patterns – if there is any – were neglected.

Nevertheless, this study confirmed the role of autoantibodies in predicting autoimmune comorbidities in T1DM and also demonstrated a way to quantify this effect.

Conflict of Interest

The authors declare that they have no conflict of interest.

Acknowledgments

Levente Kovács is supported by the János Bolyai Research Scholarship of the Hungarian Academy of Sciences.

References

1. LeRoith Derek, Taylor Simeon I, Olefsky Jerrold M. *Diabetes mellitus: a fundamental and clinical text.* Lippincott Williams & Wilkins 2004.
2. Nathan David M., DCCT/EDIC Research Group . The Diabetes Control and Complications Trial/Epidemiology of Diabetes Interventions and Complications Study at 30 Years: Overview *Diabetes Care.* 2014;37:9-16.
3. Skarstein Kathrine, Wahren Marie, Zaura Egija, Hattori Masakazu, Jonsson Roland. Characterization of T cell receptor repertoire and anti-Ro/SSA autoantibodies in relation to sialadenitis of NOD mice *Autoimmunity.* 1995;22:9–16.
4. Burton Paul R, Clayton David G, Cardon Lon R, et al. Genome-wide association study of 14,000 cases of seven common diseases and 3,000 shared controls *Nature.* 2007;447:661–678.
5. Smyth Deborah J., Plagnol Vincent, Walker Neil M., et al. Shared and Distinct Genetic Variants in Type 1 Diabetes and Celiac Disease *New England Journal of Medicine.* 2008;359:2767–2777. PMID: 19073967.
6. Somers Emily C, Thomas Sara L, Smeeth Liam, Hall Andrew J. Autoimmune diseases co-occurring within individuals and within families: a systematic review *Epidemiology.* 2006;17:202–217.
7. Somers Emily C., Thomas Sara L., Smeeth Liam, Hall Andrew J.. Are Individuals With an Autoimmune Disease at Higher Risk of a Second Autoimmune Disorder? *American Journal of Epidemiology.* 2009;169:749–755.
8. Barker Jennifer M.. Type 1 Diabetes-Associated Autoimmunity: Natural History, Genetic Associations, and Screening *The Journal of Clinical Endocrinology & Metabolism.* 2006;91:1210–1217. PMID: 16403820.
9. Green Peter HR, Jabri Bana. Coeliac disease *The Lancet.* 2003;362:383–391.
10. Barera Graziano, Bonfanti Riccardo, Viscardi Matteo, et al. Occurrence of Celiac Disease After Onset of Type 1 Diabetes: A 6-Year Prospective Longitudinal Study *Pediatrics.* 2002;109:833–838.
11. Holmes G K T. Screening for coeliac disease in type 1 diabetes *Archives of Disease in Childhood.* 2002;87:495–498.
12. Caturegli P., Remigis A. De, Rose N.R.. Hashimoto thyroiditis: Clinical and diagnostic criteria *Autoimmunity Reviews.* 2014;13:391–397. Diagnostic criteria in Autoimmune diseases 9th International Congress on Autoimmunity.
13. Kordonouri Olga, Klinghammer Albrecht, Lang Egbert B., Grters-Kieslich Annette, Grabert Matthias, Holl Reinhard W.. Thyroid Autoimmunity in Children and Adolescents With Type 1 Diabetes: A multicenter survey *Diabetes Care.* 2002;25:1346–1350.
14. Radetti G., Paganini C., Gentili L., et al. Frequency of Hashimoto's thyroiditis in children with type 1 diabetes mellitus *Acta Diabetologica.* 1995;32:121–124.
15. Castiblanco John, Arcos-Burgos Mauricio, Anaya Juan-Manuel. What is next after the genes for autoimmunity? *BMC Medicine.* 2013;11:197.
16. Triolo Taylor M., Armstrong Taylor K., McFann Kim, et al. Additional Autoimmune Disease Found in 33% of Patients at Type 1 Diabetes Onset *Diabetes Care.* 2011;34:1211-1213.
17. Catassi C., Rtsch I-M., Fabiani E., et al. Coeliac disease in the year 2000: exploring the iceberg *The Lancet.* 1994;343:200–203. Originally published as Volume 1, Issue 8891.
18. Dieterich Walburga, Ehnis Tobias, Bauer Michael, et al. Identification of tissue transglutaminase as the autoantigen of celiac disease *Nature medicine.* 1997;3:797–801.
19. Heel D A, West J. Recent advances in coeliac disease *Gut.* 2006;55:1037–1046.
20. Sollid Ludvig M. Coeliac disease: dissecting a complex inflammatory disorder *Nature Reviews Immunology.* 2002;2:647–655.
21. Swain Manorama, Swain Truptirekha, Mohanty BinoyKumar. Autoimmune thyroid disorders–An update *Indian Journal of Clinical Biochemistry.* 2005;20:9-17.
22. Hosmer D.W., Lemeshow S., May S.. *Applied Survival Analysis: Regression Modeling of Time to Event Data.* Wiley Series in Probability and StatisticsWiley 2011.
23. Therneau T.M., Grambsch P.M.. *Modeling Survival Data: Extending the Cox Model.* Statistics for Biology and HealthSpringer 2000.
24. Grambsch Patricia M., Therneau Terry M.. Proportional hazards tests and diagnostics based on weighted residuals *Biometrika.* 1994;81:515-526.
25. Durrleman Sylvain, Simon Richard. Flexible regression models with cubic splines *Statistics in Medicine.* 1989;8:551–561.
26. Royston Patrick, Altman Douglas. External validation of a Cox prognostic model: principles and methods *BMC Medical Research Methodology.* 2013;13:33.
27. Fisher Lloyd D., Lin D. Y.. Time-dependent covariates in the Cox proportional-hazards regression model *Annual Review of Public Health.* 1999;20:145-157. PMID: 10352854.
28. R Core Team . *R: A Language and Environment for Statistical Computing.* R Foundation for Statistical ComputingVienna, Austria 2014.
29. Therneau Terry M. *A Package for Survival Analysis in S* 2014. R package version 2.37-7.
30. Jr Frank E Harrell. *rms: Regression Modeling Strategies* 2014. R package version 4.2-1.
31. Feighery L, Collins C, Feighery C, et al. Anti-transglutaminase antibodies and the serological diagnosis of coeliac disease. *British journal of biomedical science.* 2002;60:14–18.

Author: Tamás Ferenci
Institute: Óbuda University, Physiological Controls Group
Street: Bécsi út 96/b.
City: Budapest
Country: Hungary
Email: ferenci.tamas@nik.uni-obuda.hu

Towards Physical Modeling of the Utilization of Ultrasound in Modern Medical Therapeutic Applications

R. Varga, K. Klapcsik, and F. Hegedűs

Department of Hydrodynamic Systems, Budapest University of Technology and Economics,
Faculty of Mechanical Engineering, Budapest, Hungary

Abstract — **In the present paper the dynamics of a single spherical gas/vapor bubble has been investigated numerically under harmonically varying pressure field (ultrasound). This simple physical model is capable of capturing the basic physical phenomena, the very high temperature and pressure produced during the oscillation of the bubble, used in various medical applications. The applied model is the Keller—Miksis equation being second order nonlinear ordinary differential equation, that takes into account the liquid compressibility. The investigated parameters are the pressure amplitude and the frequency of the sonication. The presented two-parameter map of the achievable maximum bubble wall velocity is a good indicator for the efficiency of the applications. The results show that employment of frequency below the first harmonic resonance and pressure amplitude higher than the ambient pressure is recommended.**

Keywords — **litotropsy, histotropsy, drug delivery, sonoporation, acoustic cavitation.**

I. INTRODUCTION

A novel and promising new technology started to emerge in various fields in the modern medicine is the utilization of ultrasound in medical treatments. It is well-known that during the irradiation of liquids with high intensity and high frequency ultrasound, bubbles and/or bubble clusters are formed, called acoustic cavitation. During the oscillation of such bubbles, their wall velocity can reach several thousand of m/s, which is known as the collapse phase in the literature. At the collapse site, the temperature and the pressure can be as high as 8000 K and 1000 bar, respectively [1]. After the collapse, these extreme conditions lead to the formation of strong acoustic emission, a high magnitude pressure wave or shock wave [2].

The above mentioned physical effects are the fundamentals for several therapeutic applications. The generated shock wave caused by the excited bubbles can break up kidney stones called litotropsy [3], or can ablate or remove tissues in the targeted area known as histotropsy [4]. Ultrasound is also successfully applied in drug delivery and sonoporation in which the generated pores in the cell membrane by the acoustic cavitation are used in vivo targeting of drugs encapsulated in microbubbles [5]. Finally, high intensity focused ultrasound seems to be a promising new technology in cancer therapy via the mechanical effect of acoustic cavitation [6].

The aforementioned medical applications are the main motivations to investigate a single spherical bubble under harmonically varying pressure field placed in liquid water. Although the utilization of ultrasound produces bubble ensemble, the investigation of single bubble is the main building block to understand the physical basis. The employed model is the Keller—Miksis equation, which takes into account the liquid compressibility as a first order approximation. It is a highly nonlinear, second order ordinary differential equation solved with a simple initial value problem solver build-in Matlab software environment. The main aim is to reveal the collapse-like oscillations of the bubble in the pressure amplitude – frequency parameter plane of the excitation, which can help to develop efficient operation strategies. Our results show that the application of frequency below the first subharmonic resonance of the bubble, and the pressure amplitude above the ambient pressure is highly recommended.

II. THE BUBBLE MODEL

During the oscillations of an acoustically excited bubble, its wall velocity can reach as high as $3000\ \mathrm{m/s}$. Therefore, the liquid compressibility has to be taken into account. Among the various available models, the Keller—Miksis equation is the most accurate one [7]. The mathematical form of this equation modified according to [8] is

$$\left(1-\frac{\dot{R}}{c_L}\right)R\ddot{R}+\left(1-\frac{\dot{R}}{3c_L}\right)\frac{3}{2}\dot{R}^2=$$
$$\frac{1}{\rho_L}\left(1+\frac{\dot{R}}{c_L}\right)(p_L-p_\infty)+\frac{\dot{R}}{\rho_L c_L}\frac{d}{dt}(p_L-p_\infty), \qquad (1)$$

where the dot stands for the derivative with respect to time t, $R(t)$ is the instantaneous bubble radius, c_L and ρ_L are the sound speed and the density of the liquid domain. The pressure at the bubble wall in the liquid side is p_L and far away from the bubble is

$$p_\infty(t)=P_\infty+p_A\,sin(2\pi f\,t), \qquad (2)$$

Á. Jobbágy (ed.), *First European Biomedical Engineering Conference for Young Investigators*,
IFMBE Proceedings 50, DOI: 10.1007/978-981-287-573-0_28

where P_∞ is the static ambient pressure, p_A is the pressure amplitude and f is the frequency of the excitation. The pressure inside and outside the bubble at its wall are connected via the dynamic mechanical balance written as

$$p_G + p_V = p_L + \frac{2\sigma}{R} - 4\mu_L \frac{\dot{R}}{R}. \tag{3}$$

Here, the total pressure inside the bubble is the sum of the gas pressure (air) p_G and the vapor pressure p_V. The surface tension is σ and the liquid kinematic viscosity is μ_L. The air inside the bubble obeys a simple adiabatic state of change:

$$p_G = \left(\frac{2\sigma}{R} + P_\infty - p_V\right)\left(\frac{R_E}{R}\right)^{3\kappa}, \tag{4}$$

where R_E is the size of the bubble (equilibrium radius of the unexcited system) and $\kappa = 1.4$ is the ratio of the specific heats for air.

The values of the applied parameters and material properties are summarized in Table 1. The liquid properties are calculated from the Haar—Galagher—Kell equation of state with $P_\infty = 1$ bar and $T_\infty = 25\ ^oC$.

Table 1 Values of the applied parameters and material properties

Property	Value
Ambient pressure P_∞	1 bar
Ambient temperature T_∞	25 °C
Surface tension σ	0.072 N/m
Liquid density ρ_L	997 kg/m^3
Liquid dynamic viscosity μ_L	0.00089 kg/(m · s)
Liquid sound velocity c_L	1497 m/s
Vapor pressure p_V	3166.8 Pa
Bubble size R_E	0.1 mm
Pressure amplitude p_A	0 bar - 5 bar
Excitation frequency f	3.23 kHz - 97 kHz

III. Results and discussion

The simplest and still widely used method for solving system (1) – (4) is to take an initial value problem solver with suitable initial conditions ($R(0)$ and $\dot{R}(0)$ pair) and integrate the system forward in time. After the decay of the transient solution, which needs sometimes hundreds of acoustic cycle, it converges to a stable state called attractor. By recording the properties of this long-term stable behavior, the strength of the bubble collapse and therefore the efficiency of the medical applications can be explored. Such indicators are the maximum bubble radius of the oscillation or the maximum bubble wall velocity during the collapse phase. In the following, the strength of the collapse will be systematically examined as a function of the pressure amplitude and the frequency of the excitation. In typical applications, these are the main and most easily controllable quantities. In numerical analysis, they often called as control parameters. Due to the nonlinear nature of the Keller—Miksis equation, several attractor may coexist at given excitation properties. Therefore, at each parameter pair 5 randomly chosen initial conditions were applied in order to reveal the relevant coexisting attractors. The numerical solution technique is a 4th order Runge—Kutta scheme with 5th order embedded error estimation. The employed software environment was Matlab.

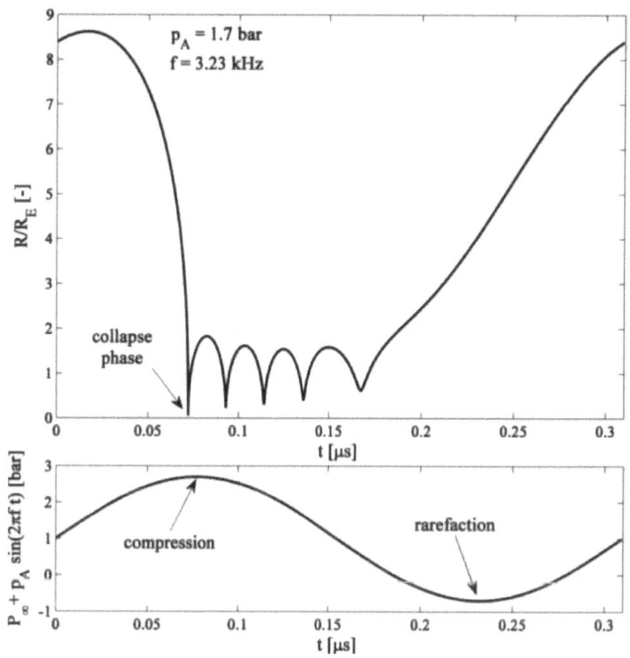

Fig. 1. Bubble radius vs. time curve in the giant response region at $p_A = 1.7$ bar and at $f = 3.23$ kHz. The lower panel represents the pressure excitation for one acoustic cycle.

Due to the time periodic pressure excitation, the simplest long-term response of the bubble is periodic, as well. An example for a typical periodic attractor at $p_A = 1.7$ bar and at $f = 3.23$ kHz is given in Fig. 1, where the relative bubble radius R/R_E is presented as a function of time. During the rarefaction phase of the ultrasonic irradiation, there is a long expansion in the bubble radius, and finally the bubble size becomes more than 8 times larger than its original size. In the compression phase, the large bubble starts shrinking followed by an extremely steep collapse with several afterbounces. Observe that after the first rebound, the local maximum of the bubble radius is much less than the absolute maximum. This is an indicator for a strong collapse, since most of the energy accumulated during the rarefaction phase is emitted into the liquid domain manifested as a strong shock wave [2]. Here, the applied frequency is well below the resonance frequency $f_0 = 32.3$ kHz corresponding to the present bubble size $R_E = 0.1$ mm. This frequency domain is called the giant response region in the literature [8].

For the strength of the collapse, the bubble wall velocity vs. time curve is more expressive shown in Fig. 2. At the time instant of the collapse, the wall velocity reach as high as 3000 m/s, which is two times greater than the sound speed in the liquid domain indicated supersonic bubble wall velocity, compare the value with Table 1. The energy loss during the first collapse is clearly seen, as the maximum velocity in the first rebound is only a fraction of its predecessor.

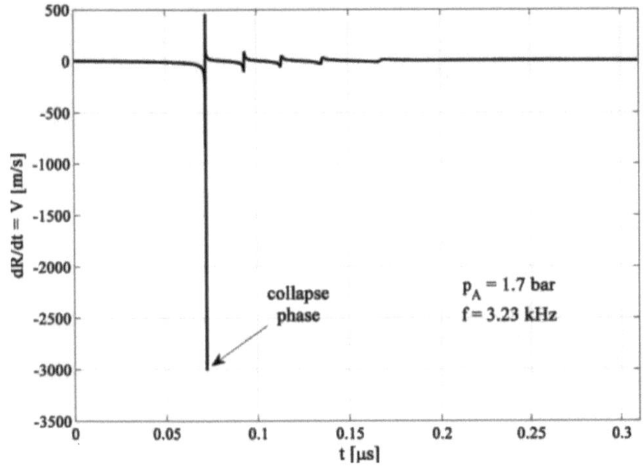

Fig. 2. Bubble velocity vs. time curve in the giant response region at $p_A = 1.7$ bar and at $f = 3.23$ kHz.

Driving the bubble at its resonance frequency $f = 32.3$ kHz and with higher pressure amplitude $p_A = 3$ bar, several changes in the behavior in the dynamics can be observed, see Fig. 3. The bubble response is still periodic; however, the period of the attractor is two times than that of the excitation. Such solution is called period 2 orbit in the language of nonlinear dynamics. In the second compression phase of the ultrasonic irradiation, a steep collapse can also be noticed indicated by the rapid change in the direction of the oscillation.

Solely from the relative bubble radius vs. time curves, the strength of the collapse cannot be compared properly. Therefore, the bubble velocity is again presented as a function of time in Fig. 4. Now, it is evident that the collapse is much weaker than in the previous case, as the achievable maximum bubble wall velocity is approximately 550 m/s, which is well below the sound speed in the liquid domain (subsonic velocity). Observe that the maximum bubble wall velocity is scaled with the maximum bubble radius. The larger the maximum radius the higher the bubble wall velocity, compare Fig. 1 – Fig. 4. Therefore, both quantities can be a good indicator for the strength of the collapse.

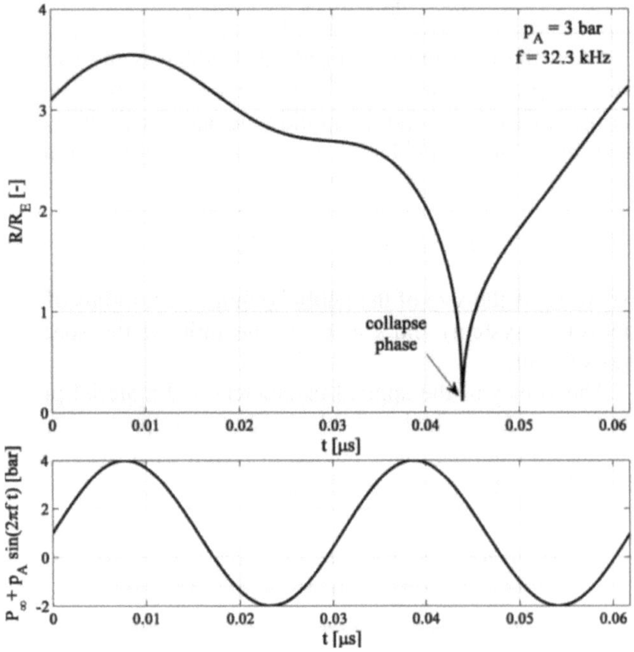

Fig. 3. Bubble radius vs. time curve at the main resonance at $p_A = 3$ bar and at $f = 32.3$ kHz. The lower panel represents the pressure excitation for two acoustic cycles.

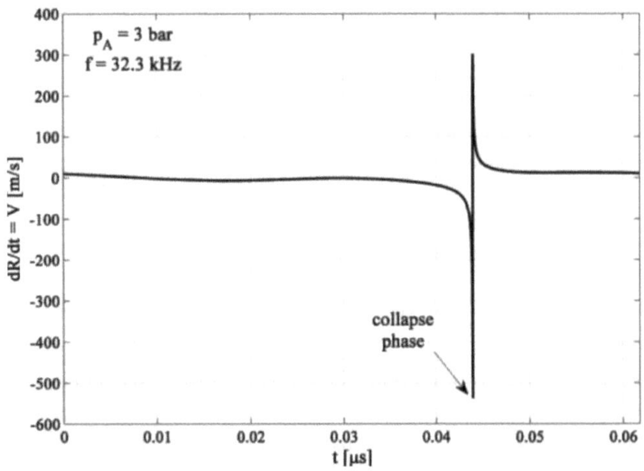

Fig. 4. Bubble velocity vs. time curve at the main resonance at $p_A = 3$ bar and at $f = 32.3$ kHz.

From the above described results, it is clear that strength of the collapse is significantly depends on the excitation parameters. The two examined parameter combination, however, gives only limited insight into these dependencies. In the following, the numerical results are extended considerably, and a high resolution bi-parametric map of the absolute maximum bubble wall velocity is presented. The applied parameter combinations during the computations, similar to those of investigated in Fig. 1 to Fig. 4, are summarized in Table 2. Again, at each parameter pair, 5 simulations were performed with random initial conditions to reveal the co-existing solutions. In case of such co-existence, the largest achievable absolute maximum bubble wall velocity was recorded out of the found multiple attractors.

Table 2 Summary of the detailed numerical parameter study

p_A	Δp_A	f	Δf
0 bar - 5 bar	0.01 bar	3.23 kHz - 97 kHz	3.23 kHz
0 bar - 5 bar	0.25 bar	3.23 kHz - 97 kHz	0.323 kHz

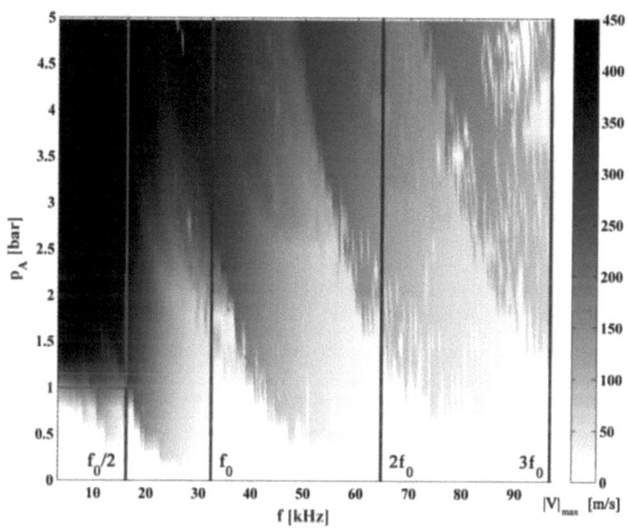

Fig. 5. Maximum absolute bubble wall velocity in m/s as a function of the pressure amplitude p_A and excitation frequency f.

The condensed representation of the detailed analysis is shown in fig. 5, as a bi-parametric contour plot of the maximum bubble wall velocities. In order to visualize the fine structure properly, the maximum velocity is limited to 450 m/s, as shown in the grayscale colormap. Therefore, in the black domain in the lower frequency region, which is the aforementioned giant response region, the bubble velocity is definitely greater than the limited value.

The giant response region is enclosed by the red lines in Fig. 5. From application point of view, it is recommended to keep the operation parameters in this domain to produce strong bubble collapse, that is, above $p_A = 1$ bar pressure amplitude (it is the ambient pressure P_∞) and below $f = f_0/2 = 32.3$ kHz excitation frequency. Naturally, this rule-of-thumb is valid for bubble size $R_E = 0.1$ mm. Parenthetically, the main resonance f_0, the first harmonic resonance $f_0/2$ and the first two subharmonic resonances $2f_0$ and $3f_0$ are denoted by the thick blue vertical lines in Fig. 5.

IV. Summary

A single spherical bubble model capable of capturing the basic physical phenomena of various, ultrasonically enhanced medical applications has been presented. The mathematical model was the well-known Keller—Miksis equation, which is a second order nonlinear ordinary differential equation. Our numerical results show that for bubble size 0.1 mm, the pressure amplitude and frequency of the ultrasonic irradiation should keep higher than 1 bar and lower than 32.3 kHz, respectively, to keep the efficiency high.

Acknowledgment

This research has been supported by the Hungarian Scientific Research Fund – OTKA, under grant no. K81621.

References

1. Brennen C E (1995) Cavitation and bubble dynamics. Oxford: University Press.
2. Minsier V, Proost J, (2008) Shock wave emission upon spherical bubble collapse during cavitation-induced megasonic surface cleaning. Ultrason. Sonochem. 15: 598—604.
3. Chaussy C, Brendel W, Schmiedt E (1980) Extracorporeally induced destruction of kidney stones by shock waves. Lancet 316: 1265—1268.
4. Xu Z, Ludomirsky A, Eun L Y et al. (2004) Controlled ultrasound tissue erosion. IEEE Trans. Ultrason. Ferroelectr. Freq. Control 51: 726—736.
5. Mitragotri S (2005) Healing ultrasound: the use of ultrasound in drug delivery and other therapeutic applications. Nat. Rev. Drug Discov. 4: 255—260.
6. Kennedy J E, Haar G Rt, Cranston D (2014) High intensity focused ultrasound: surgery of the future? Brit. J. Radiol. 76: 590—599.
7. Prosperetti A, Lezzi A (1986) Bubble dynamics in a compressible liquid. Part 1. First-order theory. J. Fluid Mech. 168: 457—478.
8. Lauterborn W, Kurz T (2010) Physics of bubble oscillators. Rep. Prog. Phys. 73: 106501.

Author: Roxána Varga
Institute: Department of Hydrodynamic Systems
Street: Műegyetem rkp. 1-3.
City: Budapest
Country: Hungary
Email: rvarga@hds.bme.hu

Author Index

Keyword Index

MIX
Papier aus verantwortungsvollen Quellen
Paper from responsible sources
FSC® C105338

If you have any concerns about our products,
you can contact us on
ProductSafety@springernature.com

In case Publisher is established outside the EU,
the EU authorized representative is:
Springer Nature Customer Service Center GmbH
Europaplatz 3, 69115 Heidelberg, Germany

Printed by Libri Plureos GmbH
in Hamburg, Germany